W9-AYN-414

BODY SCULPTING BIBLE FOR ABS

WOMEN'S EDITION

Deluxe DVD Edition

THE BODY SCULPTING BIBLE FOR ABS

WOMEN'S EDITION

Featuring the 14-Day Ab Sculpting Workouts
The Ultimate Workout Program for the Ultimate Abs

Written by:
James Villepigue

Photography by:
Peter Field Peck

Hatherleigh Press * New York

Text, Photographs, and DVD ©2007 The Hatherleigh Company, Ltd.

No part of this book may be reproduced, stored in a retrieval system, or transmitted, in any form or by any means, electronic or otherwise, without written permission from the Publisher.

Hatherleigh Press
5-22 46th Avenue, Suite 200
Long Island City, NY 11101

www.hatherleighpress.com

Library of Congress Cataloging-in-Publication Data available upon request.

ISBN 978-1-57826-265-6

Disclaimer
Consult your physician before beginning any exercise program. The author and publisher disclaim any liability, personal or professional, resulting from the application or misapplication of any of the information in this publication.

THE BODY SCULPTING BIBLE FOR ABS books are available for bulk purchase, special promotions, and premiums. For information on reselling and special purchase opportunities, please call us at 1-800-528-2550 and ask the the Special Sales Manager.

10 9 8 7 6 5 4 3 2 1
Printed in the United States of America

Dedication

I would like to dedicate this book to the most important people in my life. To my, as always, incredible mom, Nancy: I am blessed by God to be your son and I thank you for all your limitless love and support. You are an inspiration to so many mothers!

To my incredibly successful sister, Deborah: I am so proud of your strong will and your drive to succeed. You have become such a remarkable businesswoman and I am so psyched to see how far you can take it!

To my beloved dad, Jim, my best pal and navigator: I love you and miss you so much. Thank you for instilling in me your boundless love, deep emotions, and adventurous spirit. I honor you absolutely every moment of my life.

To God, again and as always, thank you, thank you, thank you!

To my very beautiful, incredibly sweet, and extraordinarily talented wife, Heather Villepigue, I love you, my baby, and I am so blessed to have you by my side. Thank you!

To the newest addition to my family: Sienna James Villepigue: You entered our world on July 1st of 2007 and our lives were immediately changed. I am so proud and blessed to be your father!

Special Thanks

Mike Mejia of Spectrum Conditioning Systems (SCS) of Port Washington, New York, provided invaluable assistance in creating this book. Without him—and the use of his *facility—The Body Sculpting Bible for Abs* wouldn't have been possible!

Peter Field Peck's outstanding photography makes our exercises clear and easy to use. Many thanks, Peter.

Ed at Context Studios for his great work on the DVD. Thank you so much!

Jason G., thanks for being the great friend you are, brother!

Thank you Andrew, Kevin, Alyssa, Andrea, and the team at Hatherleigh, for the fantastic opportunities. Great things to come!

Our book models, LoreDana Ferriolo, Mimi Kim, Igor Ladanov, Guillermo Subiela, John Williams (of SCS), and Nana Wolff were troopers during the photo shoot. Thank you!

Our DVD models, Penelope Lagos and Femi Olagoke: You were both awesome. Thank you!

Precautions

READ THIS SECTION THOROUGHLY BEFORE READING ANY FURTHER!

Always consult a physician before starting any exercise or weight loss program.

If you are unfamiliar with any of the exercises in this book, ask an experienced trainer to instruct you about proper form and execution.

The instructions and advice in this book are not intended as a substitute for medical or other professional counseling.

Custom Physiques, Inc., the editors, and authors disclaim any liability or loss in connection with the use of this system, its programs, and advice herein.

Table of Contents

INTRODUCTION 1
The Road to Gorgeous Abs

PART 1: THE SCIENCE OF ABDOMINAL PERFECTION

CHAPTER 1: Know Your Abs 9
Understanding Abdominal Anatomy

CHAPTER 2: Feed Your Abs 15
Proper Nutrition for Extraordinary Abs

PART 2: WORK YOUR ABS

CHAPTER 3: The Warm-Ups 21

CHAPTER 4: Mat Exercises 41

CHAPTER 5: Swiss Ball Exercises 63

CHAPTER 6: Medicine Ball Exercises 89

CHAPTER 7: Equipment Exercises 99

CHAPTER 8: Lower Back Exercises 117

PART 3: THE BODY SCULPTING BIBLE FOR ABS 14-DAY WORKOUTS

CHAPTER 9: The Workouts 131

ABOUT THE AUTHOR 147
RESOURCES 149

Introduction
THE PATH TO GORGEOUS ABS

Forget the starvation diets, the mind-numbing repetitions of crunches, and hour after hour spent on the treadmill. We'll help you achieve the sleek, toned abs you've always wanted, but through a more balanced, sensible approach than you've seen in the past. The result will be abs that not only drop jaws at the beach, but also leave your body feeling better and stronger than ever before. So if you're tired of run-of-the-mill ab workouts that don't deliver what they promise, get ready for something radically different!

THE **BODY SCULPTING BIBLE** FOR **ABS**

WOMEN'S EDITION

THOSE FABULOUS ABS

So just what is it about abs, anyway? I don't mean their obvious appeal; who doesn't want a flat midsection? What I can't figure out is why all the confusion. Why is it that almost everybody wants great abs, but so few of us are actually able to get them? Could it be that those chosen few who do sport taut tummies are simply more disciplined than the rest of us? Perhaps they have access to some can't-miss workout that miraculously melts away unwanted flab. Or maybe—just maybe—they've been able to filter through all the hype and misinformation about abdominal training and find a strategy that works for them. I'd put my money on the latter.

You see, when it comes to abdominal training there are no ab-solutes (pun intended). What works for your girl friends may not necessarily work for you. When you consider individual differences in the rate at which our bod-

A SPECIAL NOTE FOR WOMEN WHO ARE EXPECTING

The idea of doing abdominal work when you're pregnant is a controversial issue. Some experts suggest that all ab exercises should be avoided throughout the entire pregnancy. Others insist that certain ab exercises are not only safe, but they also (1) prevent back problems during and after pregnancy; (2) make labor—when there's lots of pushing—easier; and (3) help you recover from the pregnancy more quickly. Whether or not to do ab work when you're pregnant is a decision you should make with your doctor. I would urge you not to attempt any of the exercises in this book until you have consulted him or her.

YOU MUST REMEMBER THIS

• Starvation diets and excessive cardio work can actually slow your metabolism, making it virtually impossible to burn fat.

• It takes a combination of intensive strength training and interval cardio work to provide the foundation upon which great abs are built.

• Constantly working your abs while paying little or no attention to your lower back sets you up for possible injury.

ies burn fat, varying time commitments to working out, and different dietary habits, you begin to see why no single approach works best. Sadly though, this simple fact seems to have eluded much of the fitness industry. Cookie-cutter workouts rife with isolation exercises, endless hours of cardiovascular exercise, and a caloric intake that would barely sustain a hummingbird let alone a grown woman are too often the recommended prescriptions for a head-turning mid-section. And unfortunately, given the relentless manner in which this message has been pounded into the American psyche by both the print and electronic media, it will be difficult to stem that tide.

Much of the problem springs from the fact that in our society a sleek waistline has come to represent beauty, fitness, and good health. That's ironic because healthfully low levels of body fat, while certainly desirable, don't necessarily indicate superior overall health. And flat abdominals don't always indicate that your core is strong. Unfortunately, many people in the mainstream fitness industry continue to perpetuate the notion that attaining a fat-free midriff is akin to reaching some sort of Holy Grail.

Enough is enough! For years now there's been way too much emphasis placed on aesthetics when it comes to abdominal training. Of course, it is wonderful to have beautiful abs, but what's the point if you throw out your back trying to lift a shopping bag out of the trunk of your car or picking up a 35-pound toddler.

I wish I had a nickel for every time I saw someone with "great abs" struggle to perform simple tasks like balancing on one leg or swinging a tennis racquet properly—not to mention the ones who end up hurting themselves because their abdominals and lower back (aka the "core musculature") lack the kind of strength that is important for many actions. How is this possible, you ask? How can it be that something so visually appealing can also be so structurally unsound? Simple: Performing set after set of crunches and other exercises that isolate the abdominals—particularly when it's combined with a lack of lower back training, creates posture and strength imbalances that can lead to possible injury.

DOWN WITH ISOLATION

To fully appreciate why the traditional approach to abdominal training doesn't work you need to know only one word: *isolation.* And I don't mean doing sit-ups all alone in your living room. By isolation I mean targeting and exercising a specific muscle or muscle group to work without the assistance of others. And when it comes to abdominal training, no exercise accomplishes that better than the ever-popular crunch. Unlike its cousin, the much-maligned full sit-up, the crunch alleviates undue strain on the neck and lower back and reduces the contribution of the hip flexors. That ability to safely and effectively isolate your abs—specifically the *rectus abdominis* (see diagram on page 13)—that has made the crunch the darling of physical therapists and personal trainers alike for the past dozen years or so.

The biggest surprise isn't that all that crunching failed to produce the results people wanted; it's that this "isolation fascination," as I like to call it, continues to be so widely

THE PRE-STRETCH SOLUTION

So the traditional crunch works your abs through only about half their range of motion. The solution, however, is not to sit up a bit farther. Besides being incredibly difficult to do, coming up higher than that 30 degrees taxes the hip flexors to a large extent—not something most folks need to do given the adverse effects that tight, overworked hip flexors can have on proper posture.

The best way to increase the range that your abs have to work through (and the intensity of the resulting contraction), is to stretch your abdominals backward about 30 degrees into what I call a pre-stretch position. But bending backward 30 degrees is impossible when you're already lying on the floor. That's where the Swiss ball comes in. Besides increasing the demand on your core musculature to help stabilize your position on the ball, performing crunches and other similar exercises on the Swiss ball enables you to drop your head and shoulders back slightly and effectively pre-stretch the abdominals. But what if you don't have a ball you ask? (Don't worry, on page 42 I've described a way you can get this same effect using a common bath towel.)

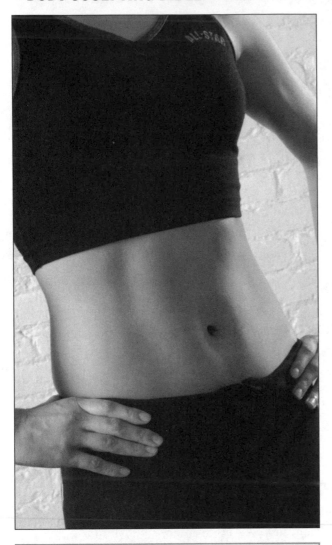

TAKE THE TOTAL BODY APPROACH

Listen up: You can work your abs until you're blue in the face, but if that is the only exercising you do, you will never get the sleek, fabulous abs you want. The metabolic demands aren't great enough to make an appreciable change in your body composition. The bottom line? there's no such thing as spot-reducing, so if you want great abs, you've got to work your entire body.

accepted. Walk into any gym and I guarantee that you'll see at least a half dozen people mindlessly crunching their hearts out. If they only knew that without making changes to their diets and engaging in total-body workouts that promote fat loss, no amount of abdominal training will miraculously melt away that spare tire. To make things worse, those folks who are working so hard on those crunches are actually promoting postural imbalances that can set them up for injuries in the future.

I'm not knocking crunches; the problem is that most people perform them to the exclusion of other important ab and back exercises. Look at the diagram on page 13 and you'll see that the major muscle of the abdominals—the *rectus abdominis*—originates at the breastbone and lowermost ribs and inserts on the pelvis. When the muscle contracts, it flexes the spine to produce an action like the one you do when you perform a crunch. The problem is that when you do a crunch in the traditional manner—by laying flat on the floor—you're working the *rectus abdominis* muscle through about only half of its range of motion, 30 degrees or so.

What it all comes down to is that lots of people do lots of different types of crunches, and each kind works the *rectus abdominis* muscle through only about half its range of motion. In the meantime, most people virtually ignore the opposing muscle group in the back (it's called the *erector spinae* group; it acts to extend the spine). What happens? Over time your abdominal wall can shorten and pull your pelvis out of alignment. That places lots of undue strain on your lower back and can wreak havoc with your posture. And for what? Doing all those reps doesn't help you burn any more fat and it doesn't give you fab. abs. Why then are so many people convinced that this is the way to great abs? Because that's what we've been trained to believe. Up until now, anyway.

STICK WITH IT!

Congratulations! You're about to embark on a new phase of your fitness training. That's the easy part. Sticking with the program can get to be a challenge. Here are some ways to maintain your motivation on your way to *supremo* abs.

1 Start with small goals that lead to larger goals. For example, if your life is very hectic, start with the small goal of doing your ab work once a week and work up to your ultimate goal of working them three times each week. As you accomplish the easier goal you'll be encouraged to keep working toward the larger goal.

2 Set attainable goals. Losing 50 pounds in one month is neither a realistic nor safe goal. Losing six to eight pounds in one month is more like it. When you set goals you can't possibly reach, you're only sabotaging yourself.

3 Reward yourself when you attain your goals. Treat yourself to a new outfit or a (sensible) dinner out with friends.

4 Take pictures! The camera never lies. Once a month take a photo of yourself and put it on the fridge or paste it into your training log. While you may notice small changes from week to week, a monthly photo will show just how far you've come.

5 Think positively. Your attitude can go a long way toward helping you achieve your goals. Think of yourself as healthy and fit. Visualize yourself as an athlete—strong and energetic.

6 Listen to your body. The better you begin to feel and look, the more tempted you may be to overdo your workouts. When your muscles start to ache more than usual, if you begin to suffer from insomnia or unusual fatigue, you might be overtraining. Lower the intensity of your workouts for a while.

It's time for a fresh start. You want great abs. You need a strong core. This book—with our Body Sculpting Bible for Abs exercises and the 14-Day Workouts—will give you both.

THE 14-DAY WORKOUTS

The 14-Day Ab Sculpting Workout is a system that takes a safe and holistic approach to ab work, enabling you to reach your goals in the minimum amount of time. Why 14 days? That's typically the amount of time that it takes most people to adopt a new habit. It's also how long it takes your body to get used to a new training scheme. Building a habit (like waking up early to workout) can be good, but it's not productive for your body to get used to a workout. Once it does, you'll stop seeing results. (For a full explanation, see *The Body Sculpting Bible for Women*. Also, changing your workout every two weeks will keep you from getting bored.

If you've been putting off getting your midsection into shape, now's the time to start. I can't promise that it'll be easy—you have to work for great abs. But I truly believe that this book will get you started. Good luck!

—*James Villepigue*

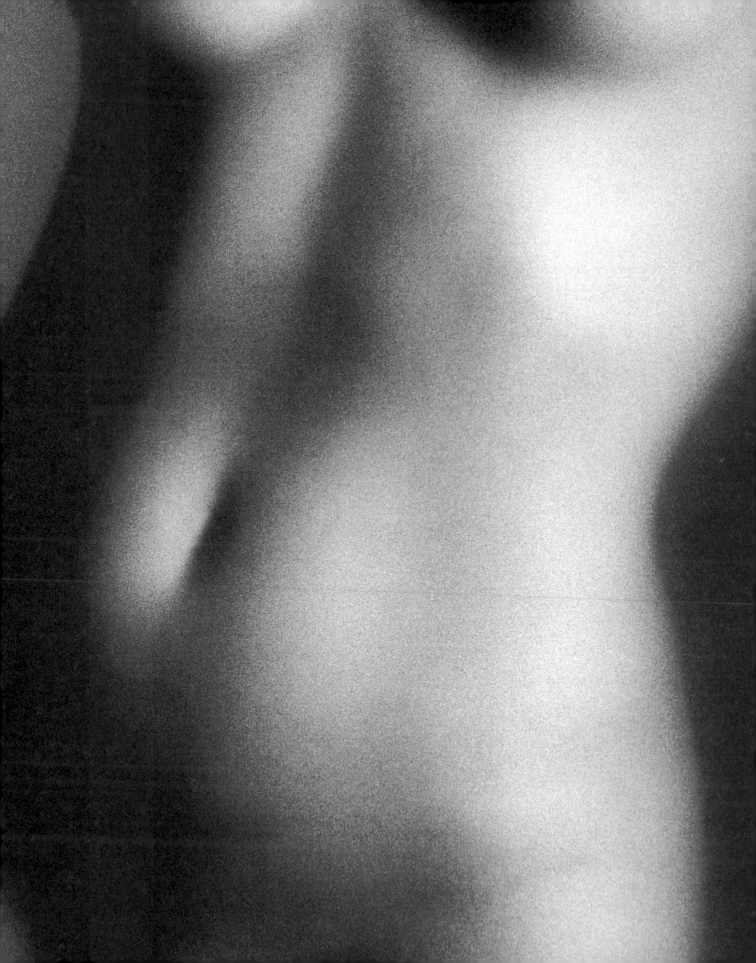

Part 1

THE SCIENCE OF ABDOMINAL PERFECTION

You want knock-out abs, the kind that turn heads and inspire envy. Well, there are three steps you'll have to take:

KNOW YOUR ABS.
NOURISH YOUR ABS.
WORK YOUR ABS.

Here in Part I we'll explore those first two steps. (The rest of the book is devoted to Step 3!) In Chapter 1 you'll learn a little about the specific muscles that make up the abs and how they work. Then, in Chapter 2, you'll learn how to eat right to get those fabulous abs.

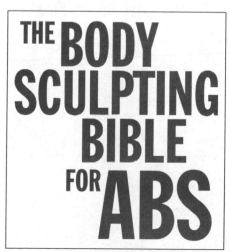

THE **BODY SCULPTING BIBLE** FOR **ABS**

WOMEN'S EDITION

EXERCISES FOR EACH MUSCLE GROUP

RECTUS ABDOMINIS

Towel Crunch
Crunch with Lateral Flexion
Slow Sit-Up
Lateral Bridge
V-Up
Knee-In
Bicycle
Swiss Ball Crunch
Swiss Ball Circle Crunch
Swiss Ball Jackknife
Swiss Ball Cobra
Swiss Ball Pass Off
Swiss Ball Crunch with Rotation
Swiss Ball Bridge
Swiss Ball Praying Mantis
Medicine Ball Kneeling Throw
Medicine Ball Overhead Sit-Up
Medicine Ball Bicycle
High-to-Low Cable Woodchopper
Low-to-High Cable Woodchopper
Slant Board Reverse Crunch
Hanging Leg Raises
Hanging Oblique Raise
High Chair Scissors
Overhead Squats
Good Mornings
Suitcase Dead Lifts
Unilateral Romanian Dead Lift

TRANSVERSE ABDOMINIS

Towel Crunch
Slow Sit-Up
Lateral Bridge
V-Up
Vacuum
Swiss Ball Crunch
Swiss Ball Jackknife

Swiss Ball Pass Off
Swiss Ball Praying Mantis
Medicine Ball Overhead Sit-Up
Cable Crunch

OBLIQUES

Crunch with Lateral Flexion
Bicycle
Swiss Ball Oblique Crunch
Swiss Ball Circle Crunch
Swiss Ball Crunch with Rotation
Medicine Ball Woodchopper
High-to-Low Cable Woodchopper
Low-to-High Cable Woodchopper
Saxon Side Bends
Hanging Oblique Raise

TOTAL ABS

Windshield Wipers
Twisting Pulse-Up
Swiss Ball Corkscrew Crunch
Swiss Ball Figure Eights
Swiss Ball Crunch with Cross Body Leg Lift
Deadlifts

BACK/ERRECTOR SPINAE

Lateral Bridge
Swiss Ball Corkscrew Crunch
Swiss Ball Cobra
Swiss Ball Bridge
Supermans
Deadlifts
Overhead Squats
Good Mornings
Suitcase Dead Lifts
Unilateral Romanian Dead Lift

Chapter 1
Know Your Abs:
Understanding Abdominal Anatomy

To get the really sexy midsection you want, you need to know where your abdominal muscles are and how they work. Then you'll better understand how to work them effectively. On the next few pages you'll discover everything you ever wanted to know about ab anatomy—and why the traditional approaches to abdominal training don't work.

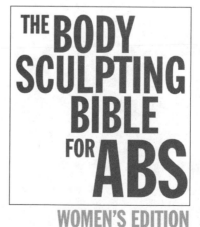

1

THE BODY
SCULPTING
BIBLE
FOR ABS
WOMEN'S EDITION

MEET YOUR ABS

How much do you really know about the structure and function of your abdominal muscles? I'd almost guarantee that you're neglecting at least one of the important ones. This short ab-natomy lesson will help you understand how your abs work—and how you can sculpt them to their full potential.

AB-NATOMY CLASS

Knowing something about the different parts of your abdomen and how they work is important. It's been my experience over the years that the more in tune people are with their bodies, the more equipped they are to push them to perform better. Knowing what muscles you're training and having a mental picture of how they're moving as they contract during an exercise helps you form the kind of mind-muscle connection that leads to more productive training. Besides which, it takes your mind off the burn some of these exercises deliver!

The abdominals are made up of a few distinct muscle groups that have a variety of different functions. Take a look at the diagram on page 13 for an illustration of what I'm talking about.

First is the *rectus abdominis,* by far the most well-known of the abdominal muscles. It's the muscle guys mean when they talk about a "six pack"—you have one, too. The *rectus abdominis* starts at the sternum and rib cage and inserts on the pubic bone. The primary job of the muscle is to flex the spine, but it also pitches in when you bend to the side (also known as lateral flexion) and rotate your trunk. Whenever you do traditional abdominal exercises, like variations of crunches and leg raises, you're primarily targeting the *rectus.*

The next muscle group is made up of the *external* and *internal obliques.* The external oblique originates on the lateral portion of the ribs and attaches to the crest of the ilium; the internal oblique originates on the crest of the ilium and fans out to attach to attach to the pubic bone and several ribs. These two muscles work in unison to help you twist and lean.

The *transverse abdominis* (TVA) lies deep

GET A CLUE ABOUT YOUR CORE

If you do any kind of working out, you've no doubt been hearing the word *core* a lot lately. *Core* is gym jargon for the lower back and abdominal muscles. The core is important for a number of reasons.

❶ It serves as the link between your upper body and lower body. So, for example, when you swing a tennis racket, you're using your abs and lower back muscles in concert to twist your torso.

❷ The core stabilizes your body during almost any movement: Bending down to pick up your shoes, running to the bus, throwing a Frisbee™, or jumping to reach a blanket from a shelf.

❸ The core protects your body during extreme exertion, like when you're lifting something heavy, whether it's a bag of groceries, a suitcase, or a child.

COUNT OUT COUNTLESS REPS

If you've read and used *The Body Sculpting Bible for Women* (and I hope you have!) you know my stand on countless reps: They don't work and in fact are counterproductive. Sets of each exercise should consist of *8 to 15 reps.* Here's why:

1 It's the range within which the output of growth hormone is maximized—growth hormone decreases body fat.

2 Performing so many reps increases blood flow to the muscles, which provides them with nutrients and helps them recover more quickly.

3 Keeping the number of reps you do in the 8 to 15 range decreases dramatically the possibility of injury since you need to use a weight that you can control to perform that number of reps.

beneath the other abdominal muscles and in fact, most people have no clue that it even exists. That's a shame, because the TVA plays a crucial role in increasing overall spinal stability and is instrumental in proper lifting mechanics. Ever heard a trainer or therapist advise someone to keep their stomach pulled in when they lift a heavy object? When you pull in your stomach you're using your TVA to reduce the likelihood of lower back injury. But despite the muscle's vital in spinal stability, most traditional ab exercises don't involve it at all.

That's right, cranking out rep after rep of crunches does little if anything to train your TVA. So besides increasing your risk of injury by creating a weak link in your core, not working your TVA can also have adverse effects from an aesthetic standpoint as well. You see, the TVA functions much like a corset, pulling your abdominal wall inward toward your spine. If trained consistently, the TVA can actually help give your waistline a more sleek, hollowed out look. Did you ever notice an individual who had little if any fat on their waist, yet still had a little paunch

sticking out over their belt? That could be the result of not specifically targeting the TVA. But don't worry: I've included several great TVA exercises in this book.

Now that you know where your ab muscles are and how they work, we can clarify one of the long-standing misconceptions about them. For example: There are no such things as "upper" and "lower" abs. The *rectus abdominis* is one long sheet of muscle that runs from your breastbone to your pelvis. When you perform almost any type of sit-up or leg raise the entire muscle contracts, if for no other reason than to help stabilize your torso. When you perform the Hanging Leg Raises (page 108), the lower part of the *rectus* and your hip flexors do the majority of the work to lift your legs toward your chest and the upper part contracts to help keep you from swinging all over the place. It's true that during some exercises, you feel the movement more in one part of your abdominal wall than another, but trust us: The entire muscle is working.

Let's review:

Your abdominals are made up of several muscle groups: the *rectus abdominis,* the

WHAT WOMEN WANT

There are some issues about which men and women will almost certainly express dissenting views: the merits of channel surfing, the excitement of shopping, and the wisdom of asking for directions, to name a few. So when it comes to working out it's no surprise that men and women often have differing agendas. Women tend to prefer a sleeker, more "toned" appearance; men usually prefer a buff, chiseled look. Occasionally you'll see a woman sporting a set of rippling abdominals; however, given the fact that women carry more body fat than men around the waist, hips, and thighs, her ability to do so is either the result of some unbelievable dedication to diet and training—or perhaps some pharmacological cheating. It's difficult (and potentially dangerous) for a woman to get her body fat low enough to achieve the kind of abdominal development that men can.

Another way in which men and women tend to differ in their approach to ab work is in their willingness to try new things. I've found that women are, by and large, more amenable to experimenting with new training methods.

I think that these contrasting views about exercise have a lot to do with the results men and women actually get from training in general and abdominal work in particular. For example, women will be far more likely to try exercises such as the Swiss Ball Bridge on page 84 and the Slow Sit-Up on page 46 once they realize that doing so will improve their ability to lift things without fear of injury. Throw in the fact that these exercises give their waistline the kind of sculpted look they're after and they're even more enthused. (Men, on the other hand, tend to shy away from exercises like these because (a) they can be difficult to perfect; and (b) they don't give you a killer abdominal burn.)

Women may be more adventurous than men when it comes to working out, but they're a lot less likely to use added resistance. Much of that probably has to do with the (outdated) belief that lifting weights leads to big, bulky muscles. The truth is that you needn't worry. Adding a little resistance to your ab exercises will not give your waistline a thick, blocky look. The bottom line: Women have a harder time building muscle than men.

Like any other muscle group, your abdominals need to be progressively overloaded to receive a training effect. But adding resistance to abs exercises should be done judiciously. You don't have to use a ton of weight, just enough so that your abs begin to fatigue toward the last few repetitions of the set. Be careful, too, that any additional weight you do use doesn't compromise your ability to do the exercise properly. So for instance, if you're performing a weighted sit-up holding an 8-pound dumbbell across your chest and have difficulty completing the range of motion, drop down to five pounds. Likewise, if the added weight doesn't provide enough of a challenge, bump it up a little. The whole idea is to force the muscles you're training to adapt to the new stimulus and become stronger. If you're not doing that, you're just spinning your wheels.

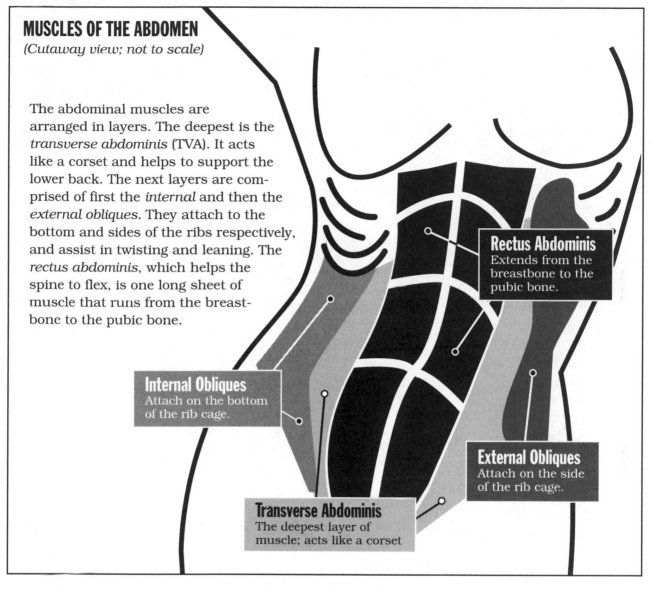

MUSCLES OF THE ABDOMEN
(Cutaway view; not to scale)

The abdominal muscles are arranged in layers. The deepest is the *transverse abdominis* (TVA). It acts like a corset and helps to support the lower back. The next layers are comprised of first the *internal* and then the *external obliques*. They attach to the bottom and sides of the ribs respectively, and assist in twisting and leaning. The *rectus abdominis*, which helps the spine to flex, is one long sheet of muscle that runs from the breastbone to the pubic bone.

Rectus Abdominis
Extends from the breastbone to the pubic bone.

Internal Obliques
Attach on the bottom of the rib cage.

External Obliques
Attach on the side of the rib cage.

Transverse Abdominis
The deepest layer of muscle; acts like a corset

external and internal obliques, and the *transverse abdominis* (TVA).

The oft-ignored TVA muscle can pull in your belly and help prevent lower back injury—*but only if you work it.*

The word *core* refers to your lower back and abdominal muscles. They form the important link between your upper and lower body. A strong core protects your body when you lift heavy objects.

There are no such things as "upper" and "lower" abs! The *rectus abdominis* is one long muscle—you cannot spot train one or the other part.

That's the anatomy lesson. Now, as you perform your ab exercises, or any exercises for that matter, concentrate on the muscles being worked and I guarantee that you'll see better results.

Chapter 2

Nourish Your Abs:
Proper Nutrition for Extraordinary Abs

If there's one thing standing between you and the willowy waistline of your dreams, it's probably a layer of fat around your middle. If you want a sexy midsection, you're going to have to eat right. But don't panic—we're not going to tell you to eat less. In fact, depending on some specific factors, you just might get to eat a little more!

2

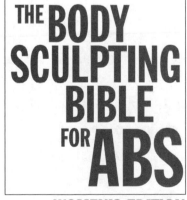

THE **BODY SCULPTING BIBLE** FOR **ABS**

WOMEN'S EDITION

GOOD NUTRITION—GORGEOUS ABS

It's the same old story: If you want really spectacular abs, you'll need to pay attention to your diet. After all, great abs don't mean anything if they're buried under a layer of flab. How much (if any) body fat you'll need to lose depends on such factors as how high your body fat percentage is when you start and what exactly you want your abs to look like. If all you're looking for is a flat tummy, you might not have to make many changes. If however, you want the kind of rippling she-devil abs that make people gawk when you wear a midriff, you're probably looking at getting your body fat down to around 20 percent.

What's the best way to lose the fat? Despite the myriad opinions, finding a method that works is a challenge. Many fat-loss programs require drastic caloric restrictions and extreme amounts of cardiovascular exercise. The problem is that most also do a pretty good job of wasting away your muscle mass in the process. Regardless of what your goals might be, losing muscle tissue is never a good idea. Losing muscle mass slows your metabolism to

---

DETERMINING YOUR DAILY CALORIC NEEDS

The first step in determining how many calories you need to consume is to estimate your Basal Metabolic Rate (BMR), which is the number of calories you need to consume each day to maintain basic body functions.

BMR = Body Weight in Pounds x 10

A 140-pound woman's BMR: 140 x 10 = 1400 calories.

That means to maintain her weight, a 140-pound woman—even if she stayed in bed all day—would need to consume 1400 calories a day.

Of course, not many of us spend the day in bed. That's why you need to add an "Activity Factor" to your BMR:

ACTIVITY LEVEL
Sedentary: BMR x .30
Moderately Active: BMR x .50
Very Active: BMR x .75

Let's say that our 140-pound woman is Moderately Active:

1400 x .50 = 700 calories

Once you know your Activity Factor, add it to your BMR, and then add another 10 percent to that total to account for calories consumed by digestion.

Again, using our 140-pound Moderately Active woman:

1400 + 700 = 2100

2100 x 1.10 = 2310 total calories *to maintain current weight.*

a crawl (during exercise and at rest)—as does decreasing your caloric intake. Is it any wonder that so many people end up confused and frustrated?

Say good-bye to all of the quick-fix training programs, "fat burning" supplements, and ridiculously low calorie diets. The best way to get results is to follow a dietary plan that will enhance your ability to build muscle and to increase your metabolic rate through intensive, total-body strength training and interval cardio work. How much you need to eat depends on a number of factors including the amount of lean mass you currently have on your body, the rate at which your body breaks down food for energy, and your daily activity level. Check the accompanying sidebar *Determining Your Daily Caloric Needs* to figure out out much you should be eating.

If you want to lose body fat, use the formula in the sidebar to determine your caloric needs and then subtract 500 calories per day from that number. This will be your new daily caloric intake. Even if it's more calories than you're already consuming, don't worry. You need to get your metabolism revving by getting it out of starvation mode. As long as those calories are coming from the right kind of sources (more on that later) and you're doing the workouts in *The Body Sculpting Bible for Women,* you won't gain fat. Of course, increasing your caloric intake means you'll have do more than just work your abs for 15 minutes three or four times per week. (See *Get Your Affairs in Order,* page 23)

Here are some broad guidelines to help you on your road to a lean figure

Once you know your daily caloric needs, divide that amount into five or six small meals. This will give you a constant influx of protein for muscle building and keep your blood sugar levels stable, giving you sustained energy throughout the day.

THE NOT-SO-GRAND OBSESSION

Like any other muscle group, the abs should regularly receive some direct stimulation. You could argue that because of the crucial role they play in proper posture and many other aspects of human movement that the abs should receive far more attention than muscle groups such as the chest, biceps, or calves.

But—and this is a big but—you should not focus on your abs to the point of obsession, especially if that obsession ends up sabotaging other aspects of your training program. For really great abs (and overall body strength) you'll also need to engage in some form of total-body training and cardio program to help build muscle and boost your metabolic rate.

For weight loss, I suggest that 35 to 40 percent of daily calories come from protein, 35 to 40 percent from carbohydrates, and 20 to 30 percent from fat. (These figures will vary from person to person.)

Consume most of your carbohydrates early in the day (when most people are more active), then start tapering your carb intake and upping your protein and fat consumption.

Limit your intake of white flour, white rice, white potatoes, pasta, fruit juices, and other "fast acting" carbohydrates. They're easy for your body to break down into blood sugar and cause a sharp rise in your insulin production. High insulin levels impede your body's ability to burn fat. So, although many of the foods listed above contain no fat, consuming them when you'll be less active can increase your chances of storing the calories as fat. Instead, opt for whole grain breads and ccreals, sweet potatoes, and brown rice whenever possible.

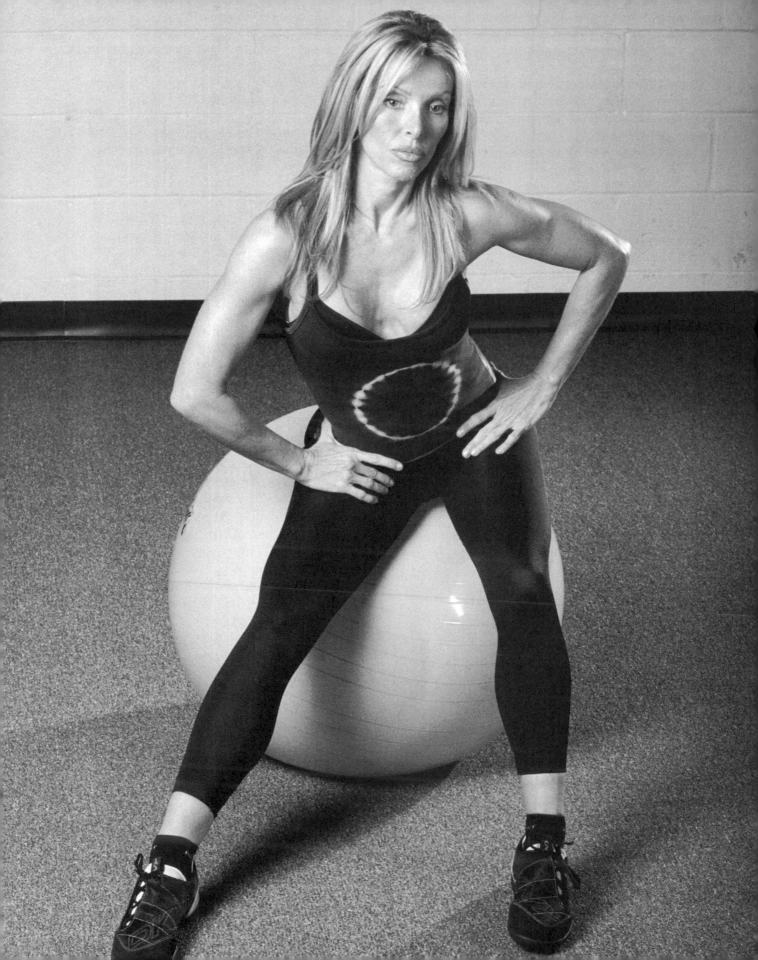

Part 2

WORK YOUR ABS

It's time to get down to business. In this section you'll find out how to effectively warm up your core before you dive into the Ab Sculpting exercises. We've divided those into several sections: Mat Exercises, Swiss Ball Exercises, Medicine Ball Exercises, and Equipment Exercises.

THE BODY SCULPTING BIBLE FOR ABS

WOMEN'S EDITION

Chapter 3
The Warm-Ups

3

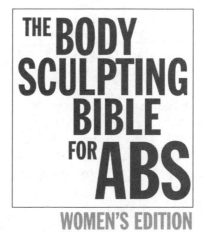

WARMING UP TO YOUR WORKOUT

Before you can get started on your new gut-busting exercises, you need to warm up. One of the easiest ways to injure yourself is to jump into any type of exercise program when your body is "cold." ("Cold" doesn't necessarily mean reduced body temperature, but rather that your body is attempting to go from a resting state into intensive physical activity.) To do that without risking of injury, you need to engage in some form of progressive, large muscle group activity to help raise your core temperature and increase blood flow to your working muscles and connective tissues. This increase in temperature and blood flow helps lubricate your joints and readies them for the kinds of repetitive motions they'll carry out during your workout. It also makes for the easier transmission of nerve impulses that stimulate your muscles to contract.

A general warm-up prepares your entire body for increased physical activity. The most common warm-ups usually involve such activities as running, cycling, rowing, or various forms of calisthenics. Typically these activities are done for 5 to 10 minutes, or until you break a light sweat. This is the way that most people warm-up prior to exercising—or should I say most people who actually bother to warm-up in the first place.

But as valuable as a general warm-up is, it's not enough to prepare your body for the demands of strenuous training. You also need to perform a specific warm-up to familiarize your muscles and central nervous system with the types of movements they'll be asked to execute during your workout.

By performing some of the same movements that you'll be doing during your actual training session (albeit at a much lower level of intensity), you can bring about more forceful and efficient muscle contractions than you could had you simply knocked out 5 minutes on a treadmill. An example of a specific warm-up would be performing a light set of bench presses with an empty barbell before moving on to more challenging loads. This "wakes up" your central nervous system, allowing it to better synchronize the movement sequence it will experience later under more intense conditions. Think of it as a dress rehearsal; the more familiar your central nervous system is with the exercise beforehand, the more efficiently it can recruit your muscle fibers to contract to produce force.

But how do you perform a specific warm-up for your abs when in many instances you'll be using only your body weight for resistance? All you really need to do is stimulate them with some low intensity contractions that involve such movements as spinal flexion and rotation. Exercises like pelvic tilts, lying on your back and bringing your knees to your chest, and unweighted rotational movements will all help prepare you for the types of exercises in this book. You'll also want to throw in some form of spinal extension and lateral flexion, examples of which I've included. The key is to keep the intensity of these drills low. The idea is to warm these muscles up, not fatigue them to the point where it will compromise your workout performance.

IT'S A STRETCH

After warming up, many people do some form of static stretching for the muscles they're about to train. In static stretching, you bring the muscle or muscles in question into a stretched position and then hold it for anywhere from 30 seconds to two minutes. This is done to relax the muscle and increase its range of motion. The problem with static stretching is that holding your muscle in the stretched posi-

GET YOUR AFFAIRS IN ORDER

Like I've said, besides watching how you eat, you'll need to get your workouts in order. I'm not talking about your ab workouts. What I mean here is the training you do for the rest of your body. To get the lean look you're after, you need to combine regular resistance training with interval cardio work in addition to your ab workouts. There are a couple of ways to do this. Depending on your schedule and individual training goals you can opt to (1) do two or three total-body workouts per week; or (2) choose a more traditional split routine in which you train different muscles on different days. Whichever you choose, be sure to incorporate lots of big compound lifts such as squats, dead lifts, bench presses, and rows. For detailed descriptions of how to safely perform these exercises, as well as complete workout routines, check out *The Body Sculpting Bible for Women*.

As for your cardiovascular workouts, the phrase to remember is interval training. Normally when you see someone doing cardio they're usually going about it at a nice steady pace. You very rarely see someone alternating between a minute or so of near all-out work like sprinting and a minute or so of a more relaxed pace, like a jog or a fast walk. That's too bad because that approach will get you fitter, faster and is a more effective way to burn fat. What's that? You always heard that lower intensity cardio work burned more fat? Nope. Working at a lower intensity may burn a greater *percentage* of calories from fat; however, all else being equal, you'll burn more total calories and fat calories by working at the higher intensity. Not to mention the fact that because it's much more metabolically taxing, interval training also offers a much more potent cardiovascular stimulus.

tion sends it a signal to relax. That may be fine at the end of a workout, but you don't want your muscles to relax just before your workout, when they will have to contract forcefully. The goal of a post warm-up stretch is to prime your muscles for the increased activity to come, not put them to sleep.

I'm not advocating that you skip stretching before you work out. If you're too tight, you'll have difficulty performing the exercises correctly and increase the chances of getting injured. The trick is to increase your muscles' range of motion and ready them for the strenuous work to come. The best way to do this is through dynamic stretching. Rather than hold the muscle in a stretched position until it begins to relax, in dynamic stretching you quickly, yet smoothly, bring the muscle into a stretched position and then immediately release it. This sequence of stretching and releasing is then repeated several times. The result is that the muscle "opens up" a bit more each time you stretch it. Dynamic stretching is a far more effective method for preparing a muscle group for the specific demands of the workout and has often been linked to improved athletic performance.

Take a look at the warm-ups on the following pages and choose three or four to do each time you do your ab workouts. If you train your abs at the end of your regular strength workouts, these exercises on their own should serve as adequate preparation. But if you give your abs priority by either training them before or on a separate day from your strength workouts, be sure and engage in a five to 10 minute general warm-up period prior to beginning these drills.

Alternating Knees to Chest

Here's one of my favorite full-body warm-ups. It's especially effective for loosening and stretching your upper and lower back as well as your abdominal muscles.

TECHNIQUE AND FORM

1 Lie on your back on an exercise mat with your arms at your sides and your legs stretched straight out in front of you.

2 Bend one knee, pull it into your chest, and then hug it around the shin.

3 Hold this position for one second and then immediately release it back to the starting position as you simultaneously repeat the same sequence with the opposite leg.

4 Continue until you've performed 6 to 10 reps with each leg.

TRAINER'S TIPS

✪ Especially when you're warming up, it's important not to force your joints beyond their range of motion. It might be tempting to squeeze your leg too tightly, but don't force it.

✪ As you pull your knees to your chest, press your lower back into the ground and gently pull your belly button in toward your spine.

✪ If you have tight knees, you can hug your legs under your lower legs, around your thighs.

✪ If your lower back feels tight, go back to your general overall warm-up to increase blood flow to the area.

Alternating Knees to Chest

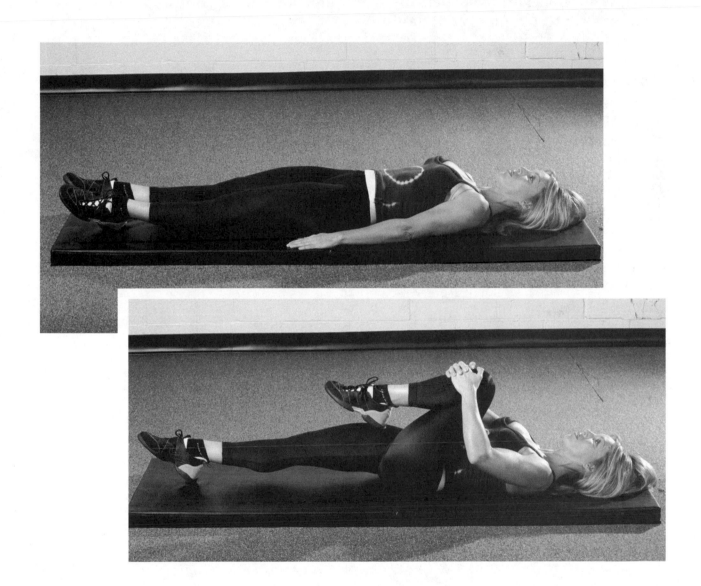

The Roll

Not only is this exercise especially helpful for loosening your upper and lower back, but it's fun to do, too.

TECHNIQUE AND FORM

1 Sit up on the exercise mat with your feet flat on the floor, your knees bent and almost together, and your chest as close to your thighs as you can get them.

2 Now tuck yourself into a ball: Keeping your heels as close to your rear end as possible, hug your arms around your upper shins and grab hold of one of your wrists.

3 Pull your abdominals in tight to your spine and tuck your chin to your chest. Exhale as you gently roll back until your shoulder blades make contact with the floor.

4 Inhale as you roll back up, contracting your abs and returning to the starting position. Continue for 8 to 10 reps.

TRAINER'S TIPS

⊛ Some people tend to hold their breath during an exercise, but it's important to keep breathing. Pay attention to the rhythm of your breaths.

⊛ As with the previous exercise, if your back or knees feel tight, go back to your general warm-up before proceeding.

The Roll

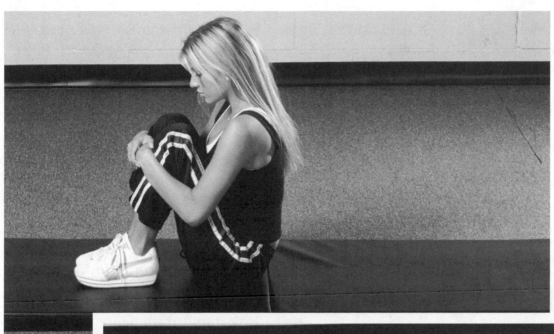

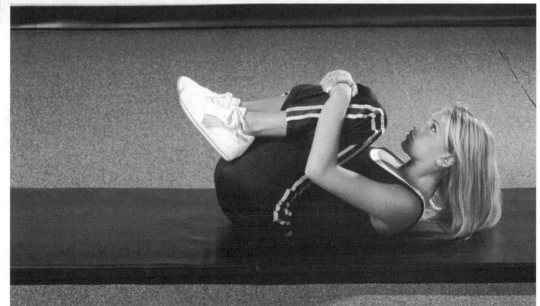

Pelvic Tilt

This exercise will help you find and maintain your "neutral spine"—a position in which your back is stable and less prone to injury. This warm-up also gently moves the spine and stretches the lower back.

TECHNIQUE AND FORM

1 Lie on your back with your feet flat on the floor and your knees bent at a 90-degree angle. In this starting position you should have a very slight arch in your lower back, but no more than you would if you were standing up.

2 Inhale deeply and then exhale as you pull your belly button into your spine. Flatten your lower back into the exercise mat and tuck in your buttocks, pressing them up toward the ceiling.

3 Hold the position for five to 10 seconds and then repeat. Continue for 10 to 12 reps.

TRAINER'S TIPS

✪ Think of your pelvis as a bowl of water; As you contract your abs and glutes you're attempting to spill the water onto your stomach.

✪ Breathe during the exercise and remember to keep your lower back pressed into floor throughout.

✪ This exercise can also be performed by itself to alleviate sore back muscles.

Pelvic Tilt

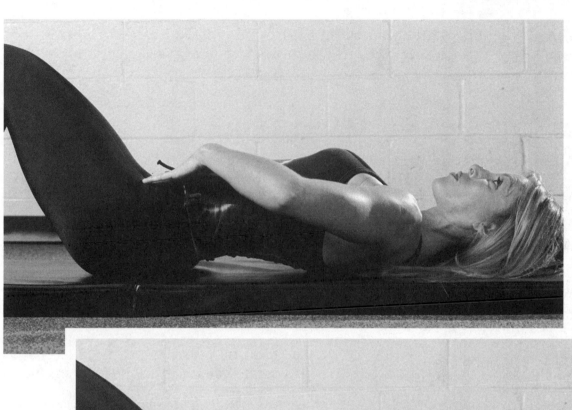

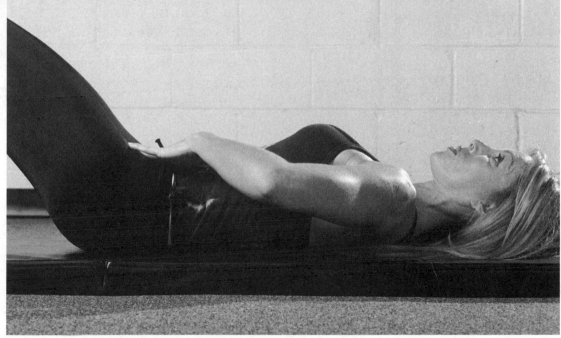

Press Up

This is the classic ab stretch and warm-up. You may have heard it referred to by another name, the Cobra. When you perform this exercise, remember that in the topmost position it's important to keep your hips on the floor and not to lock your arms.

TECHNIQUE AND FORM

1 Lie flat on your stomach with your legs straight out behind you and your arms next to you, as if you were going to do a push-up.

2 Slowly lift your torso by extending your arms until your chest and abdominals are off of the floor. Open your chest. In the top position your arms should be straight but not locked.

3 Hold the position for a moment and then repeat for 8 to 10 reps.

TRAINER'S TIPS

● When you're in the topmost position, your pelvis should still be in contact with the floor.

● Never force this stretch; come up only as far as is comfortable—both for your abs and your back muscles.

● Keep your lower back and buttocks relaxed during this stretch.

● If at any point you experience pain in your lower back, stop the exercise.

● If you're not flexible enough to extend your arms for this stretch, you can modify the exercise by coming up onto your bent elbows.

Press Up

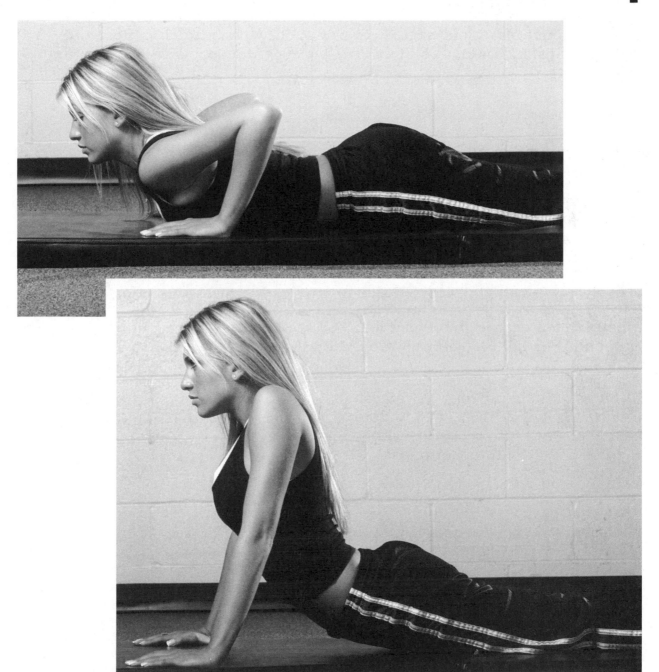

Rotational Stretch

The Rotational Stretch is a terrific warm-up for your buttocks, hips, and your lower back. Again, don't force the movement, especially if you're just starting out.

TECHNIQUE AND FORM

1 Lie on your back with your knees bent and your feet flat on the floor.

2 With your arms held down to your sides, lift and bend your left leg and place the outside of your left ankle against the outside of your right knee.

3 Keeping both shoulder blades completely in contact with the ground at all times, allow the weight of your left leg to pull your right leg over toward the floor.

4 Get as close to the floor as you can before bringing your legs back to the starting position and repeating with the other side. Continue for 6 to 8 reps on each side.

TRAINER'S TIPS

It's important that you keep your upper back and shoulders in contact with the floor at all times during this exercise to avoid lower back strain.

You can vary this warm-up by interlacing your fingers behind your head rather than holding your arms out to the side.

Rotational Stretch

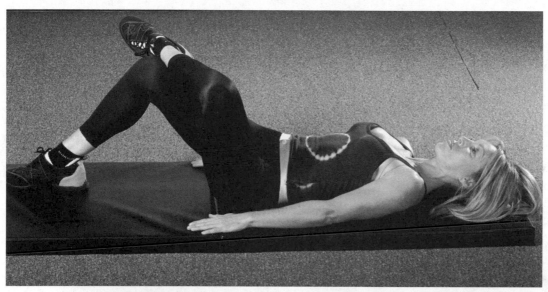

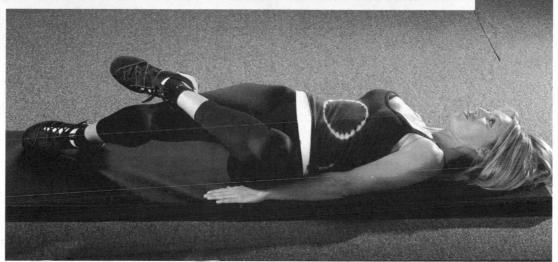

The Angry Cat

Despite its fearsome name, the Angry Cat stretch is terrific for maintaining and restoring range of motion in the back. It also encourages proper posture.

TECHNIQUE AND FORM

❶ Get down on all fours on the exercise mat. Position your hands directly below your shoulders and your knees directly below your hips. Relax your neck.

❷ With your back flat, inhale deeply, and pull your stomach in.

❸ Exhale and round your back toward the ceiling like an angry cat. In the topmost position your chin should be tucked to your chest and you should be pulling your abs in toward your spine as much as possible.

❹ Inhale as you drop your back to the starting position and repeat. Continue for 8 to 10 reps.

TRAINER'S TIPS

✪ If you've been diagnosed with ruptured disc, you should not do this warm-up.

✪ You can modify this exercise slightly by arching your back in the starting position. Let your back gently sag to the floor, then inhale deeply, pull your stomach in, and round your back.

✪ In addition to helping you warm up, this exercise is a terrific TVA conditioner.

The Angry Cat

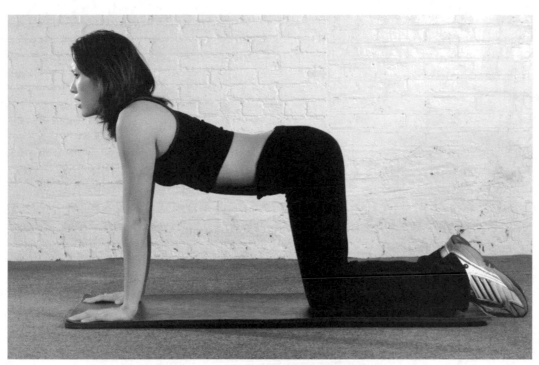

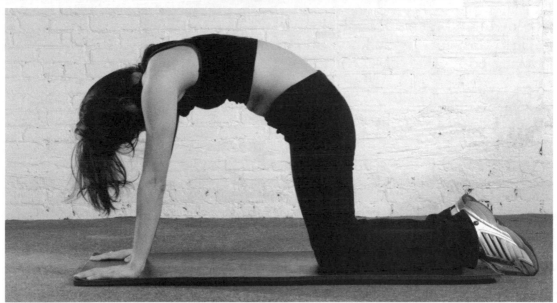

Swiss Ball Pelvic Tilt

Grab a Swiss ball for the next two warm-ups. This one focuses on your TVA and hips. One of the challenges of doing any exercise on a Swiss ball is that you need to balance yourself as you perform the exercise. This warm-up also keeps the pelvic muscles flexible, which helps lessen the chance of experiencing back pain.

TECHNIQUE AND FORM

1 Sit on a Swiss ball with your legs about shoulder width apart and feet flat on the floor. Your legs should be bent at a 90-degree angle. Place your hands on your hips or at your sides.

2 Keeping your torso as erect as possible, move the ball slightly forward by pulling your belly button to your spine and rolling your glutes underneath your body.

3 Slowly and smoothly roll the ball back to the starting position and repeat.

4 Continue for 12 to 15 reps.

TRAINER'S TIPS

✪ Swiss balls are available in many different sizes. For best results, choose a ball that is large enough that your legs are bent at a 90-degree angle when you sit on it.

✪ During this exercise, your upper body should stay in proper alignment; don't roll or shift with the movement of your lower body.

Swiss Ball Pelvic Tilt

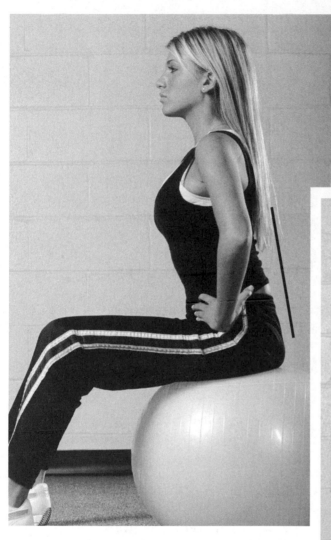

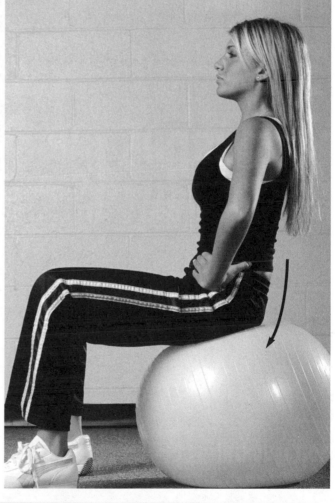

Swiss Ball Figure Eights

As with the Swiss Ball Pelvic Tilts on the previous pages, the Seated Figure Eights will help you to create and maintain flexibility in your pelvis. It also warms up your hips and your legs.

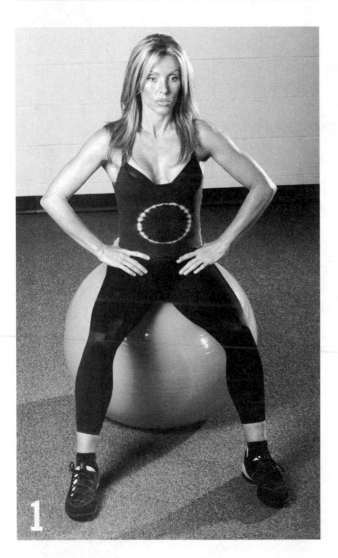

TECHNIQUE AND FORM

❶ Sit on the Swiss ball with your legs about twice your shoulder's width apart and feet flat on the floor. Your legs should be bent at a 90-degree angle.

❷ Roll your right hip forward diagonally toward your right foot, and then very smoothly arc the same hip around and toward your right rear. Next, move your hip back toward your left foot, and then back towards your left rear.

❸ Continue smoothly in this figure eight pattern for 5 to 6 reps before changing directions to the other side.

TRAINER'S TIPS

✪ Just as in the previous exercise, it's important that you not move your upper body with your lower body. Keep it as steady as you can.

Swiss Ball Figure Eights

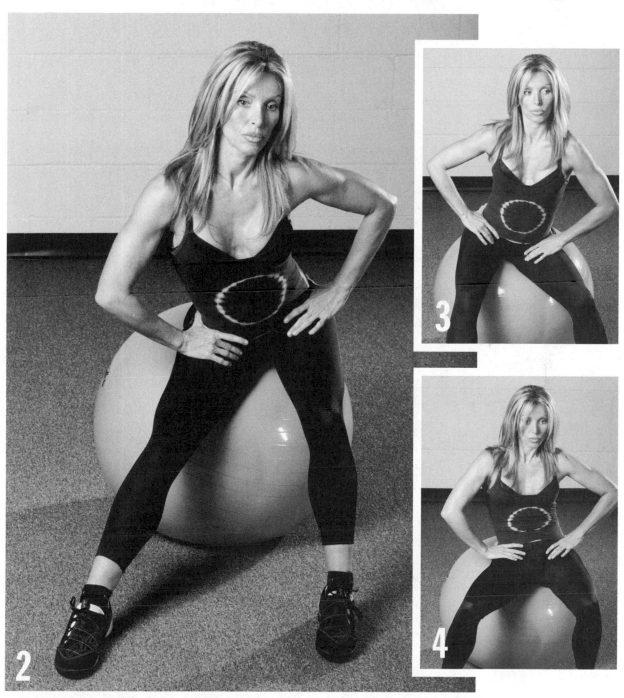

Chapter 4
Mat Exercises

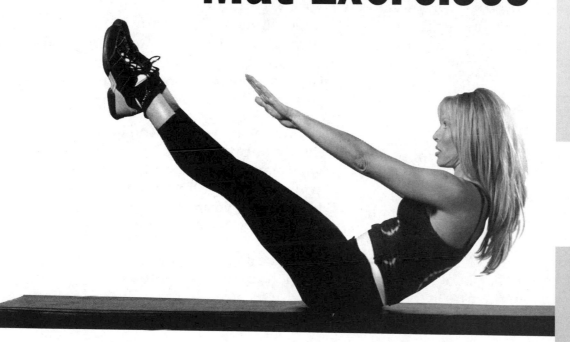

There are a number of terrific abdominal exercises you can do with nothing more than a simple exercise mat. Sure, it's nice to have access to lots of fancy equipment, but as long as you have a mat and are able to perform the types of exercise described in the pages that follow, you can give your abs an awesome workout. In fact, you could go so far as to say that many of the exercises featured here will give your abs a much better workout than they'd get on some of the fanciest gym machines. To get the most out of them though, you'll have to follow our exercise descriptions to a tee.

THE **BODY SCULPTING BIBLE** FOR **ABS**

WOMEN'S EDITION

4

Towel Crunch

By now you know that the traditional crunch doesn't work the abs through their full range of motion. The Towel Crunch helps eliminate that problem by placing the abs in a pre-stretch position, thus allowing them to contract more forcefully.

TECHNIQUE AND FORM

1 Fold a medium-size bath towel in half lengthwise and then roll it into a tube.

2 Lie on the floor with your knees bent and your feet flat on the floor. Place the rolled towel beneath you, just above the small of your back.

3 With your hands held lightly behind your head, exhale and lift your shoulder blades off the floor by crunching your rib cage toward your pelvis.

4 When your shoulder blades and upper back are a couple of inches off the floor, pause momentarily before *slowly* lowering yourself back down to the starting position.

5 Repeat for the desired number of reps.

TRAINER'S TIPS

Concentrate on pulling your abdominals toward your spine throughout the movement. This will activate the *transverse abdominis* (TVA) and protect your lower back, especially in the prestretch position.

Make sure your hands are only lightly supporting your head. Clasping your hands tightly and tugging on your head to pull yourself up takes focus off of your abs and places unnecessary strain on your neck.

Exhaling as you execute the crunch further activates the TVA and produces a more forceful contraction.

Towel Crunch

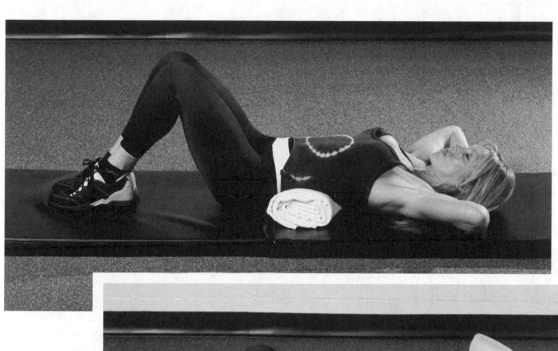

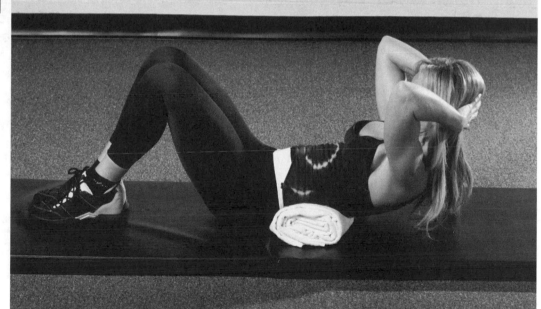

Crunch with Lateral Flexion

The Crunch with Lateral Flexion is effective on two levels: It keeps your entire abdominal wall under constant tension while really hitting your obliques.

TECHNIQUE AND FORM

1 Lie flat on the mat with your knees bent and feet flat on the floor.

2 With your hands held lightly behind your head, lift yourself into a crunch position. Don't arch your back; keep your lower back flat on the mat.

3 Holding your torso a couple of inches off the floor, bring your right armpit down toward your right hip.

4 Once you've gone as far as you are able, hold the position and squeeze your right oblique before slowly returning to the starting position and executing the same movement toward your left side.

5 Repeat for the desired number of reps.

TRAINER'S TIPS

⊗ Remember: Hold your hands *lightly* behind your head. Don't mistake just bending your neck forward for completing the exercise.

⊗ The key is to this exercise is to keep the movement completely lateral. Avoid crunching your opposite arm across your body.

⊗ Be sure that you don't allow your torso to lower as you bend laterally. Keep your shoulder blades a couple of inches off the floor throughout the entire exercise.

Crunch with Lateral Flexion

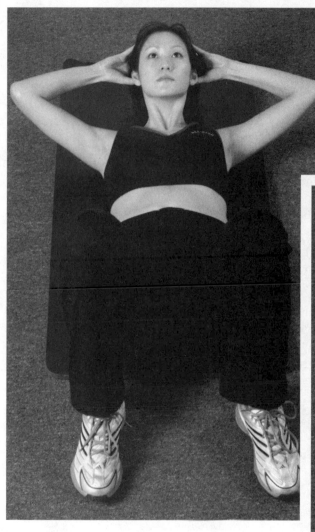

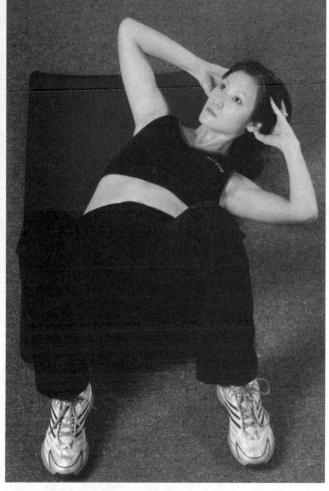

Slow Sit-Up

Despite the fact that they've been all but outlawed by many trainers and rehabilitation professionals, the sit-up remains a safe and effective exercise as long as you follow two pieces of advice: *First, do not anchor your feet under anything (like a barbell or sofa);* and second, *don't use momentum to throw yourself up off the floor.*

By not anchoring your feet, you (1) dramatically reduce the involvement of your hip flexors; (2) make your abs work much harder; and (3) reduces the chance of neck and lower back injury.

TECHNIQUE AND FORM

❶ Begin by lying on your left side on the exercise mat. Your shoulders, hips, and knees should be stacked directly over each other.

❷ Place your left forearm on the ground, perpendicular to your torso.

❸ Pulling your belly button into your spine, push your left forearm into the floor as you lift your torso and legs off the mat.

❹ In the topmost position you should be resting on the lateral portion of your left foot and your left forearm, with your right oblique in line with the rest of your torso.

❺ Lower yourself back to the starting position.

❻ Repeat for the desired number of reps before switching sides.

TRAINER'S TIPS

✪ Avoid using momentum to throw your hips up into the air; that will decrease the training effect of the exercise.

✪ Be sure that the rib cage of the working side doesn't sag toward the floor; keep the bottom oblique tucked up tight into the body.

✪ This exercise can also be done statically: Get into the finish position and hold it for 30 to 60 seconds.

Slow Sit-Up

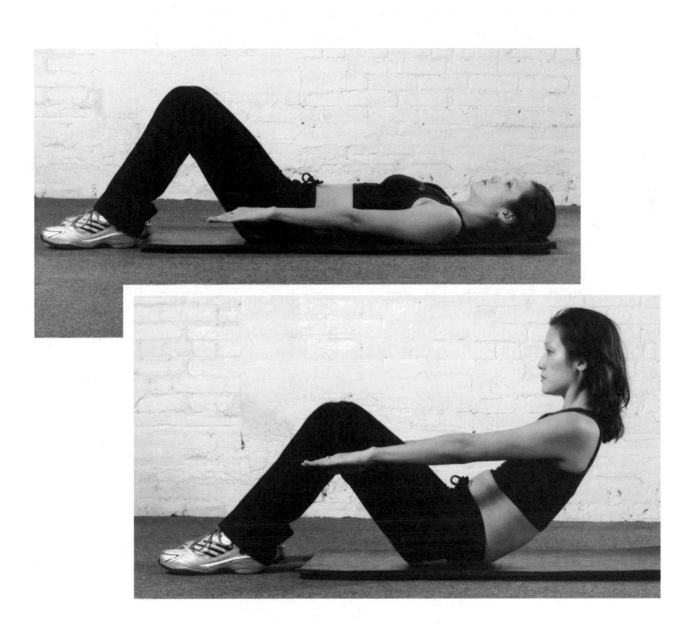

Lateral Bridge

Don't be fooled, the Lateral Bridge may look easy, but this killer exercise is terrific for increasing your abdominal strength and stability.

TECHNIQUE AND FORM

1 Begin by lying on your right side with your shoulders, hips, and knees stacked directly over each other.

2 Place your right forearm on the ground, perpendicular to your torso.

3 Pulling your belly button into your spine, push your right forearm into the ground as you lift your torso and legs off the mat. In the topmost position you should be resting on the lateral portion of your right foot and right forearm, with your right oblique in line with the rest of your torso.

4 Lower yourself and repeat for the desired number of reps before switching sides.

5 Repeat for the desired number of reps.

TRAINER'S TIPS

In this exercise—as in many of the others—momentum make make the exercise easier, but it greatly reduces the training effect. So avoid using momentum to throw your hips up into the air.

Be sure that your rib cage on the working side doesn't sag toward the floor; keep the bottom oblique tucked up tight into your body.

This exercise can also be done statically for 30 to 60 seconds.

Lateral Bridge

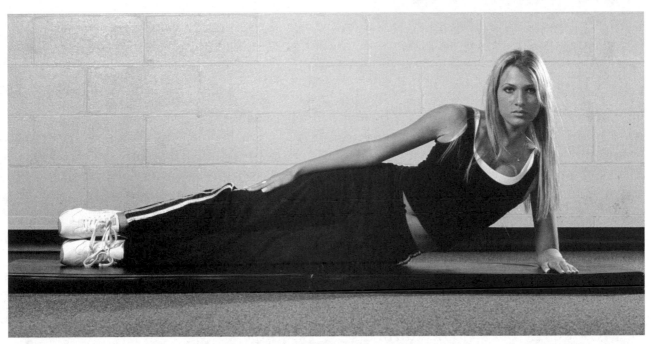

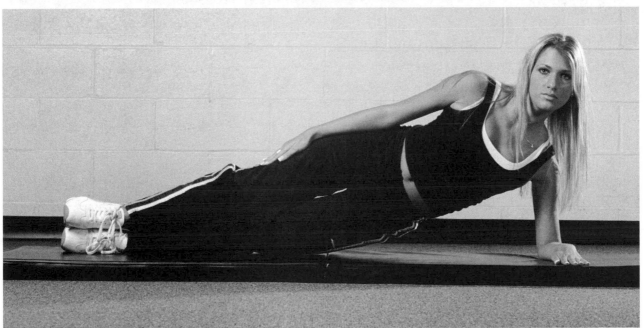

V-Up

This is a very difficult exercise. In fact, the vast majority of people I work with have to work up to it. So take your time, and don't attempt the V-Up until you're ready.

TECHNIQUE AND FORM

1 Lie on your back with your arms extended straight out behind you and your legs extended straight out in front of you.

2 Pulling your abdominals toward your spine, quickly lift your arms and legs off of the floor (at the same time) until your body forms a V.

3 Hold that position momentarily before lowering back to the starting position.

4 Repeat for the desired number of reps.

TRAINER'S TIPS

Although you need to perform the lifting phase of this exercise quickly, avoid using that momentum to heave your legs and upper body off the ground. Concentrate on using your abs to generate the necessary power.

Try to coordinate the movement as best as you can. Lifting one body segment more than or before the other will make it even more difficult to perform the exercise.

V-Up

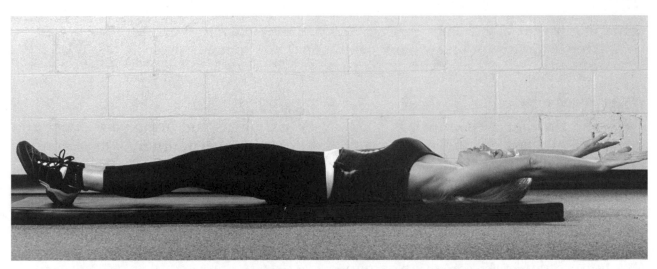

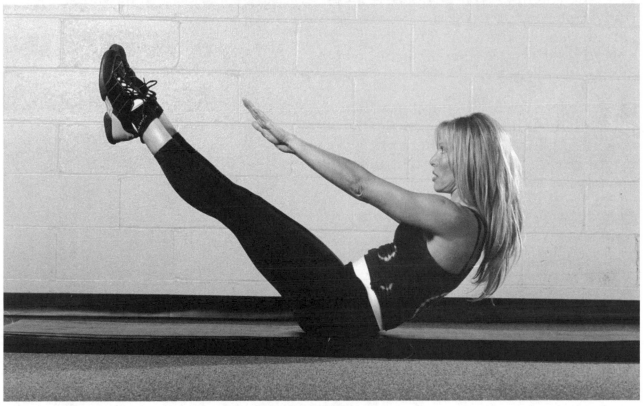

Knee-In

This is another advanced exercise that you may have to work up to. Also, if you have a history of lower back problems, take special care.

TECHNIQUE AND FORM

1 Sit on the mat with your legs stretched out straight in front of you and your arms at your sides.

2 Lean backward to the point at which you begin to feel your abdominals working to hold you in the position.

3 Once you're in that position, draw your thighs in toward your chest while simultaneously drawing your chest toward your thighs (keep a slight bend in your knees as you do this).

4 Once you reach the point at which your thighs and chest are practically touching, pause for a moment or two before returning to the starting position.

5 Repeat for the desired number of reps.

TRAINER'S TIPS

⊕ Exhale as you bring your chest and thighs together to intensify the contraction.

⊕ Keeping your arms out to your sides will help your balance. For a more challenging exercise, hold your arms overhead as you perform the exercise.

Knee-In

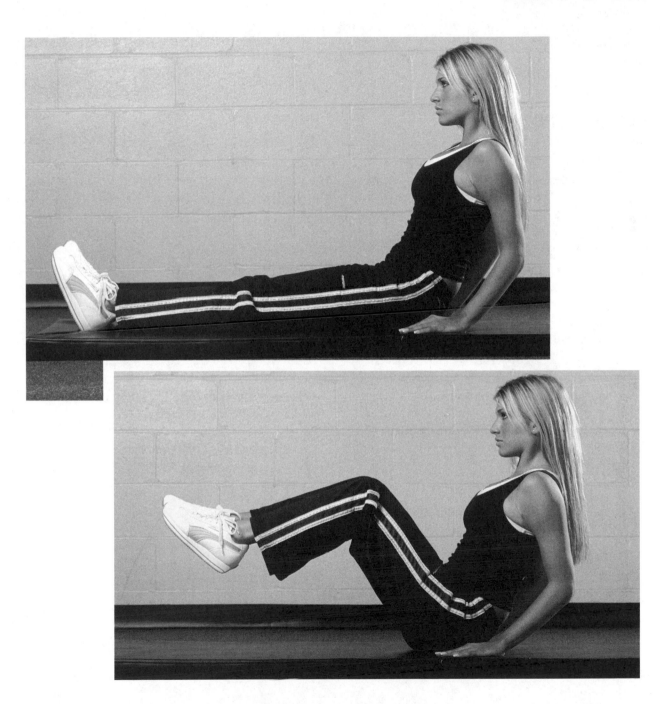

Windshield Wipers

These are great for increasing your rotational strength, but there are definitely better ways to get rain off your windshield!

TECHNIQUE AND FORM

1 Lie on your back with your arms extended out to your sides and your legs extended upward with your feet together and soles of your feet pointing at the ceiling.

2 Keeping your abs pulled into your spine, slowly lower your legs to one side and toward the floor.

3 Get your legs as close to the floor as your flexibility allows before using your abs and obliques to pull them back up to the starting position and then over to the other side.

4 Repeat for the desired number of reps.

TRAINER'S TIPS

◆ Keep the opposite shoulder blade in contact with the mat as you lower your legs to either side. Allowing your shoulder blade to come off the ground reduces the effectiveness of the exercise.

◆ Avoid using bouncing at the transition point of each repetition to generate movement in the opposite direction.

◆ Keep your belly button pulled into your spine throughout the movement. Allowing your lower back to arch excessively can result in injury.

◆ For a slightly easier version of the same exercise, repeat the movement with your knees bent at a 90-degree angle.

Windshield Wipers

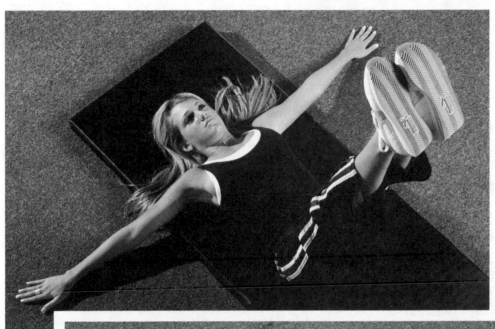

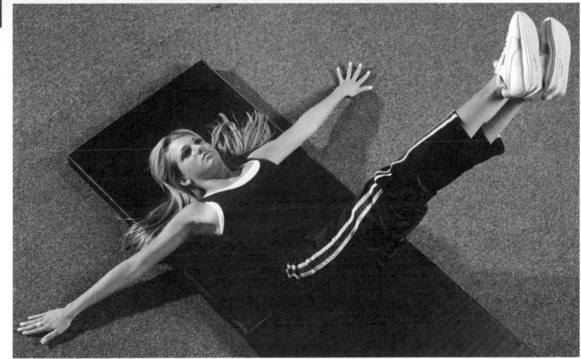

Twisting Pulse-Up

Although the range of motion may be small in this exercise, I promise you that the abdominal contraction is quite intense. Beginners beware!

TECHNIQUE AND FORM

1 Lie on your back with your legs extended up toward the ceiling and over your hips. Place your hands, palms down, at your sides or under your tailbone.

2 Keeping your legs as straight as you can, slowly lift your lower body a couple of inches off the ground by pulling your belly button toward your spine and contracting your abs.

3 At the same time, try to twist your lower body slightly by contracting your obliques and pulling your right hip up toward your right armpit.

4 Repeat for the desired number of reps.

TRAINER'S TIPS

◆ Avoid pushing off with your hands to get your lower body moving up off the floor. Concentrate on your abs.

◆ Try not to move your legs back toward your head; lift them straight up over your hips.

◆ Initiate the obliques twist by pulling your hips toward your armpit. Avoid spinning only your feet at the top of the movement.

◆ Lift and lower yourself in a slow, controlled manner. If you aren't able, you may need to work up to this one.

Twisting Pulse-Up

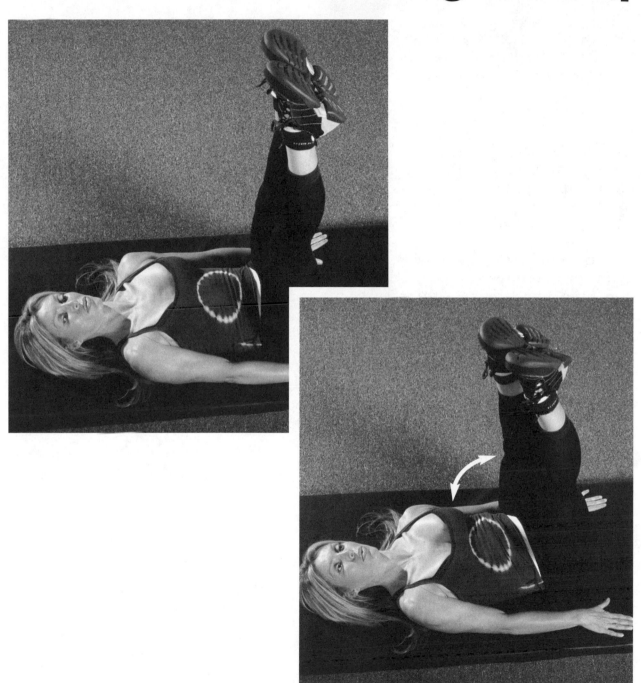

Bicycle

Okay; I admit that this exercise may look kind of hokey, but the Bicycle can actually be a very effective abdominal exercise, provided of course, that you do it properly. In fact, a recent study found that the Bicycle creates more muscle activity than any other exercise.

TECHNIQUE AND FORM

1 Lie on your back with your hands held lightly behind your head and your legs bent at a 90-degree angle over your hips.

2 With your elbows held back and out of your peripheral vision, begin by crunching across your body as you bring your opposite knee in toward your chest.

3 At the same time, extend the opposite leg and twist your torso so that the opposite elbow ends up behind you.

4 Immediately switch directions and crunch to the opposite side, bringing in the other knee.

5 Repeat for the desired number of reps.

TRAINER'S TIPS

Try to keep your lower back pressed into the floor throughout the exercise. Don't allow your back to arch excessively as you extend your legs.

Keep your elbows back and out of sight; allowing them to pull together reduces the amount of torso rotation necessary to get the most out of the exercise.

Try to keep the extended leg off the floor; allowing it to drop close to the floor increases the likelihood that you'll arch your back.

Bicycle

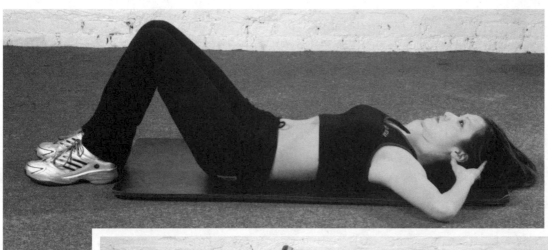

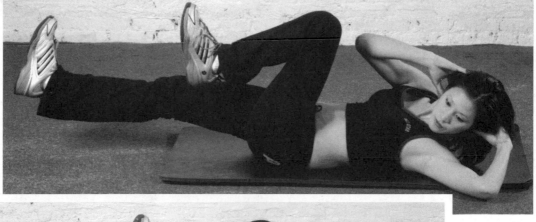

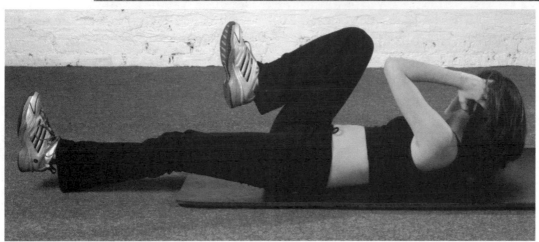

Vacuum

Here's another terrific exercise for targeting the TVA and for relaxing your entire body. Just be sure and concentrate on blowing all of the air out of your lungs to intensify the contraction.

TECHNIQUE AND FORM

1 Stand up straight with your back slightly arched and your arms at your sides.

2 Inhale as deeply as possible and then exhale, blowing out every last ounce of air from your lungs.

3 As you do so, round your back like an angry cat by pulling your belly button to your spine and dropping your chin to your chest.

4 Once you've blown out all the air, hold the position for a moment or two and breathe through pursed lips for another 6 to 10 seconds.

5 Inhale, extend your spine, and repeat for the desired number of reps.

TRAINER'S TIPS

✪ You can activate your *transverse abdominis* by pulling your belly button to your spine as you exhale. Simply blowing out your air won't do that.

✪ This exercise can be done on all fours and from a kneeling position, as well.

Vacuum

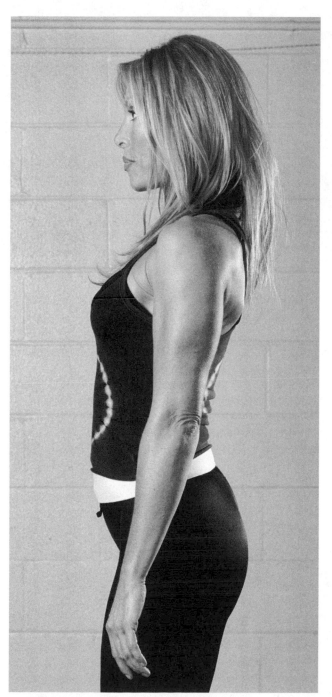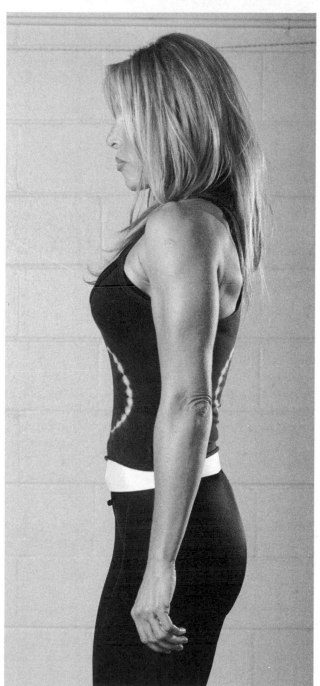

Chapter 5
Swiss Ball Exercises

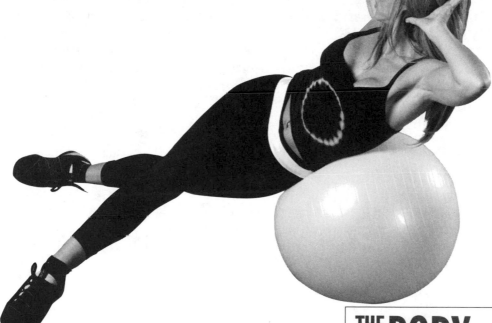

THE BODY SCULPTING BIBLE FOR ABS

WOMEN'S EDITION

5

I think of the Swiss ball as a wolf in sheep's clothing. It looks harmless enough—it's even kind of cute. But the Swiss ball is one of the most effective and intense abdominal training tools to come around in years. Besides allowing you to work through a full range of motion, the Swiss ball requires you to recruit more stabilizer muscles, thus making any exercise performed on one far more demanding.

Swiss Ball Crunch

The great thing about working with the Swiss ball is that it's unsteady. Yes, that's a good thing, because your abs are forced to work hard to steady your position. The ball also allows you to work through a more complete range of motion by placing the abs in a pre-stretch position to start the movement.

TECHNIQUE AND FORM

1 Lie back on a Swiss ball so that your head is resting on the ball and your back conforms to it. Keep your hips slightly lower than your torso and bend your knees at a 90-degree angle.

2 With your hands held back behind your head, use your abs to lift your upper back a couple of inches off the ball as you crunch your rib cage toward your pelvis.

3 Contract your abdominals and hold the position for a moment or two before lowering yourself back to the starting position.

4 Continue for the desired number of reps.

TRAINER'S TIPS

⊗ Don't pull on your head and neck to initiate your lift off the ball. Besides potentially causing injury, it reduces the training effect of the exercise.

⊗ Exhale and pull your abs toward your spine as you execute the crunching motion.

Swiss Ball Crunch

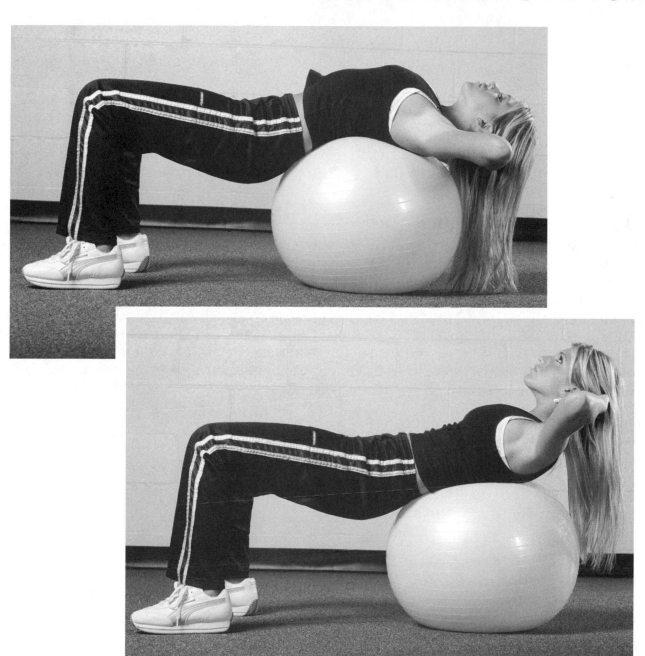

Swiss Ball Oblique Crunch

Once again, the increased range of motion provided by the Swiss ball makes this a more productive exercise than the usual oblique crunch.

TECHNIQUE AND FORM

1 Lie sideways on the Swiss ball so that only your right hip and the right side of your rib cage are in contact with it.

2 Place your hands lightly behind your head and scissor your legs so that your right leg is in front of you and your left leg is behind you.

3 Lift your upper body laterally (sideways) off the ball. In the topmost position your abs should be pulled into your spine with your torso flexed laterally toward your left hip.

4 Hold the position momentarily before lowering yourself back to the starting position.

5 Repeat for the desired number of reps before switching to the other side.

TRAINER'S TIPS

⬥ The focus here should be on initiating the contraction by bringing your top armpit toward your top hip.

⬥ You can make the exercise more challenging by extending your arms overhead or perhaps even holding a light medicine ball.

⬥ If you find that you are unable to steady yourself on the ball, use a wall to help you. Set the ball up about three feet from the wall and then prop your feet against it to perform the exercise.

Swiss Ball Oblique Crunch

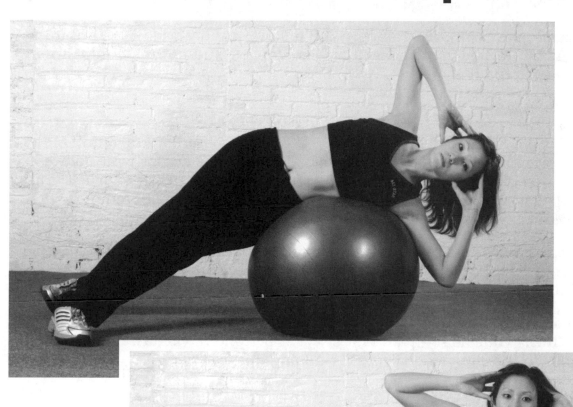

Swiss Ball Circle Crunch

This exercise starts like the standard Swiss Ball Crunch (page 64)—but it has an added twist: In this exercise, rather than coming straight up, you're arcing your torso over the ball.

TECHNIQUE AND FORM

1 Lie back on a Swiss ball so that your head is resting on the ball and your back conforms to it. Keep your hips slightly lower than your torso and bend your knees at a 90-degree angle.

2 With your hands held behind your head, lift your left shoulder blade off the ball diagonally toward your left.

3 Once you've gone as far left as you can, start lifting your torso up and laterally across to the right side of your body.

4 When you've gotten all the way to your right, lower your shoulder blades back down to the ball and repeat by starting on your right side and working toward your left.

5 Repeat for the desired number of reps.

TRAINER'S TIPS

✪ Try not to initiate the lift off of the ball by working across your body; when going to your left your left arm and shoulder blade should move first.

✪ To get the feel of the arcing motion, when going from one side to the other think of drawing a rainbow on the ceiling with your chest.

✪ Keep your elbows back and out of your peripheral vision while you're doing this exercise.

Swiss Ball Circle Crunch

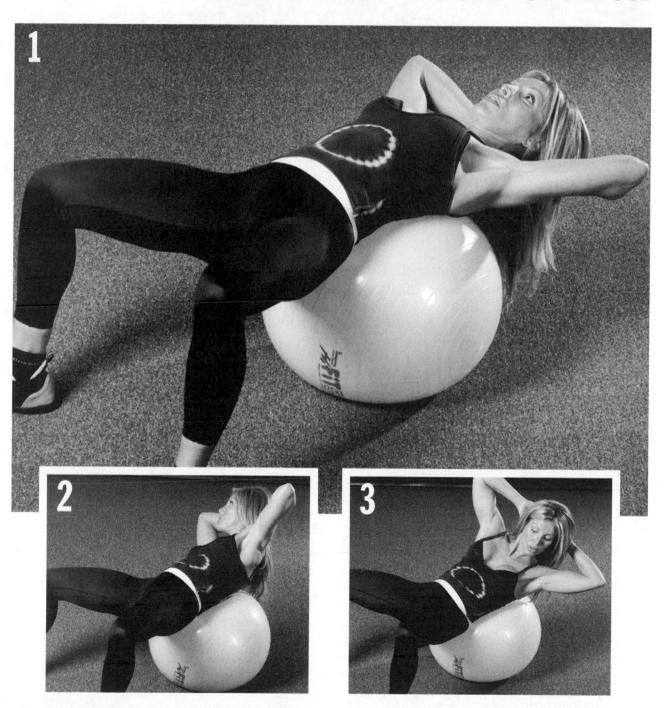

Swiss Ball Corkscrew Crunch

This crunch is really tough, so those of you who suffer from lower back discomfort may need to work up to this one

TECHNIQUE AND FORM

1 Start in the same position as for the Swiss Ball Oblique Crunch (page 68). This time however, gently twist your upper body so that for the starting position you're draped over the ball facing the floor.

2 Use your spinal erectors and oblique muscles to initiate a lift up and off the ball.

3 Once you've reached the midway position of the lift rotate your torso as much as you can so that at the top of your torso is facing forward with your abs in a crunched position.

4 Repeat for the desired number of reps.

TRAINER'S TIPS

● Perform this exercise in a controlled manner; avoid abrupt twisting or jerking movements.

● Be sure to keep your abs pulled into your spine throughout the movement to avoid potential strain to your lower back.

● If you're having trouble balancing yourself, you can brace your feet on a wall as you do this exercise.

Swiss Ball Corkscrew Crunch

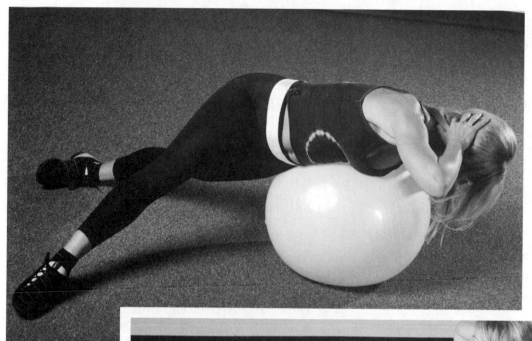

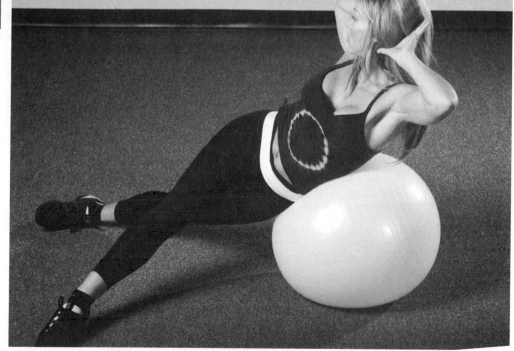

Swiss Ball Jackknife

This exercise is definitely not for beginners. You need adequate upper body strength to stabilize your position on the Swiss ball.

TECHNIQUE AND FORM

1 Begin by getting into a push-up position with your feet and lower legs resting on the Swiss ball and with your hands on the floor approximately shoulder width apart.

2 Pulling your abs in toward your spine, slowly pull your legs toward your chest by bending your knees and lifting your hips into the air.

3 At the same time, exhale and round your back as much as possible to work your abs.

4 After holding the top position for a moment or two, slowly straighten your legs and bring the ball back to the starting position.

5 Repeat for the desired number of reps.

TRAINER'S TIPS

In both the starting and finishing position of each rep proper positioning is critical. To avoid strain to the lower back, keep your abs pulled in and your glutes held tight to minimize the arch in your lower back. Allowing your abs to relax and your back to arch excessively can place tremendous strain on the back.

Concentrate on using your abs and hip flexors to pull the ball toward you.

Lift your rear end high into the air and round your back as much as possible to get maximal stimulation out of your abs.

Use a slow, controlled negative to bring the ball back to the starting position; avoid letting it roll away from you quickly.

Swiss Ball Jackknife

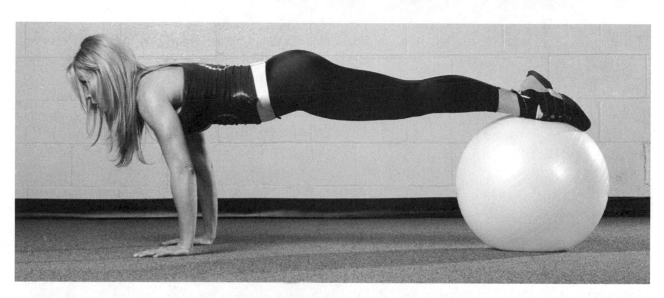

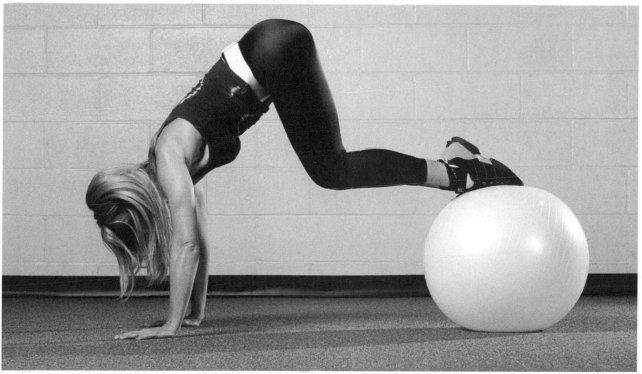

Swiss Ball Figure Eights

This is an *extremely* difficult exercise so be sure to use caution. Don't be discouraged if it takes you quite a while to work up to it.

1 Begin by getting into a push-up position with your feet and lower legs resting on the Swiss ball and your hands on the floor approximately shoulder width apart.

2 Pull the ball in toward your right armpit.

3 Once you're in the tucked position, stay there and begin to move the ball in a figure 8 pattern: Work the ball over to your left armpit using a small arcing motion and then, using your abs to control the speed of the ball, roll it out on a slight angle to your right. Still holding your abs tight, work the ball over to your left in a slight arc.

4 Repeat for the desired number of reps.

TRAINER'S TIPS

✪ Keep your abs pulled to your spine throughout the exercise.

✪ Try to use your abs, not your legs, to control the ball's path throughout the range of motion.

Swiss Ball Figure Eights

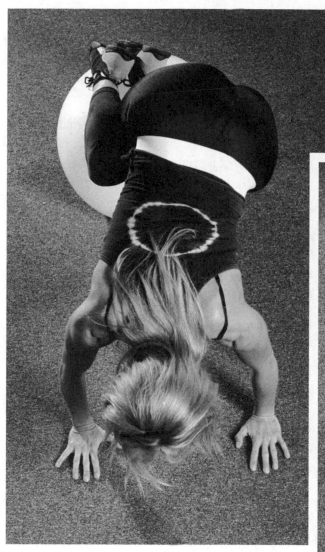

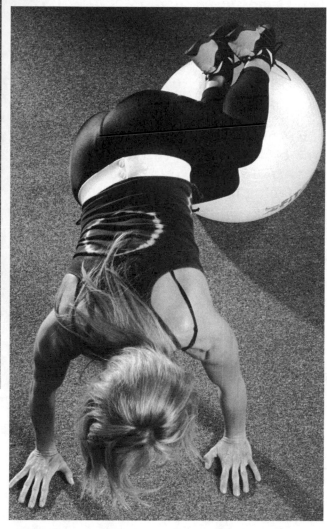

Swiss Ball Cobra

Here's another really tough one for those spinal erectors. Just as with the Swiss Ball Crunch the increased range of motion increases the difficulty level of the exercise.

TECHNIQUE AND FORM

1 Lie face down on a Swiss ball so that your chest and abdominals are in contact with the ball and your legs are straight out behind you, with only the balls of your feet touching the floor. Allow your upper body to curl over the ball and hold your arms out to your sides and bent at 90-degree angles.

2 Uncoil your spine and lift your torso off the ball. As you do so, rotate your arms so that your forearms go from facing behind you at the bottom of the movement to facing in front of you at the top.

3 At the top of the movement your back should be extended with your head, shoulders, and chest lifted off the ball and your arms rotated and even with your head.

4 Lower yourself back to the starting position by returning your arms to your sides as you allow you spine to round over the ball.

5 Repeat for the desired number of reps.

TRAINER'S TIPS

⊗ Be careful not to use momentum to lift your torso up and off of the ball. Instead slowly uncoil your spine until your back is completely straight.

⊗ Avoid completely relaxing your abs and going into extreme hyperextension when you're in the topmost position. Doing so can place undue strain on your lower back.

⊗ Keep your head pulled back in line with your spine as you extend.

⊗ Avoid jutting your chin forward as you lift.

⊗ You can make the exercise even more challenging by holding a pair of light dumbbells.

Swiss Ball Cobra

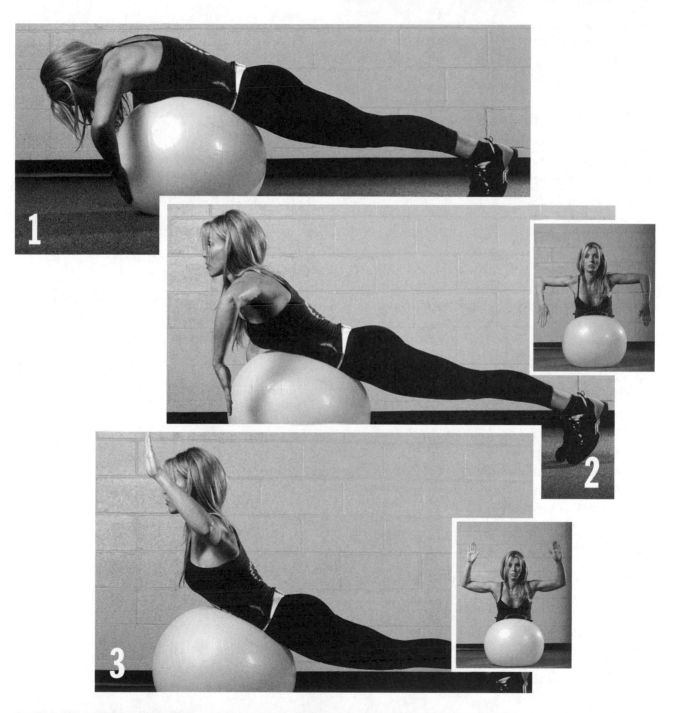

Swiss Ball Pass Off

Don't trust your eyes on this one. It might look like child's play, but if you perform it correctly, it's an ab-solute killer.

TECHNIQUE AND FORM

1 Lie on your back with your arms outstretched behind you and your legs extended up and directly over your hips.

2 Holding a Swiss ball in your hands, crunch up, lifting your shoulder blades off the floor, and place the ball between your feet. You're now holding the Swiss ball with your feet.

3 While staying in the crunch position—and leaving your arms outstretched— lower your legs as close to the floor as possible without straining your lower back.

4 Hold that position momentarily before using your abs and hip flexors to bring the ball back up and passing it to your hands.

5 Lower your arms and repeat for the desired number of reps.

TRAINER'S TIPS

As you lower your legs toward the floor, be sure your abs are pulled into your spine. That will minimize the arch in your lower back.

Make sure to lift your shoulder blades off the mat when you reach for your feet.

Initiate the arm and leg lift-offs in a controlled manner by contracting the abdominals. Avoid using momentum to propel the ball upward.

Swiss Ball Pass Off

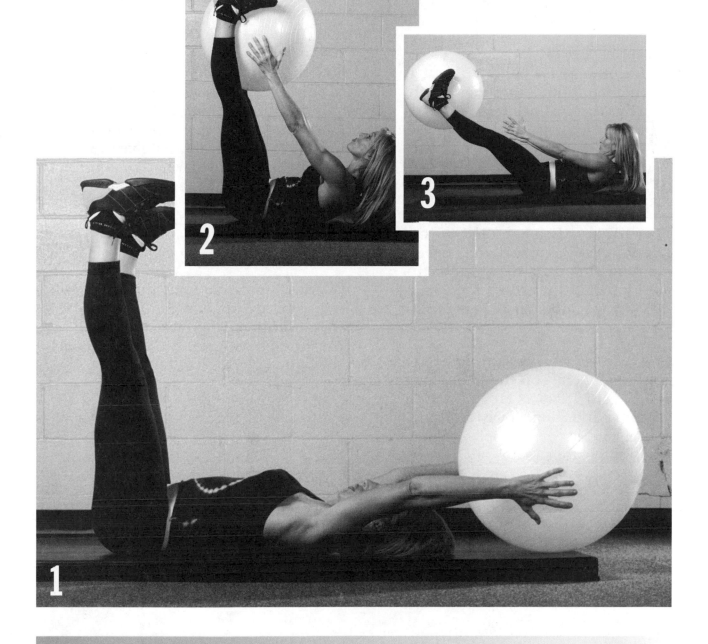

1

2

3

Swiss Ball Crunch With Rotation

Yet another Swiss ball crunch! As you can see, the ball is an extraordinarily versatile piece of equipment that offers almost endless opportunity to work your abs.

TECHNIQUE AND FORM

1 Lie on a Swiss ball with your feet on the floor about shoulder width apart and your knees bent at 90 degrees.

2 Making sure your hips are lower than your chest, lie back and allow your back to conform to the ball.

3 With your head cradled in your hands to help support your neck and elbows held out to the sides, crunch your rib cage toward your pelvis by lifting your shoulder blades off the ball.

4 Once your shoulder blades are a couple of inches off the ball, slowly rotate your torso as far to the right as possible and then slowly return to the center and lower yourself back to the starting position.

5 Repeat the same sequence on the other side and continue for the desired number of reps.

TRAINER'S TIPS

✪ Throughout the rotation be sure to keep your elbows back and beyond your peripheral vision. Allowing your elbows to pull across the head puts strain on your neck and gives you a false sense of how far you're actually rotating.

✪ Try not to lower out of the crunch position until you've completed the entire rotation.

✪ You'll find that your hips need to shift slightly to allow for complete torso rotation. Therefore, be extra careful to maintain your balance on the ball.

Swiss Ball Crunch with Rotation

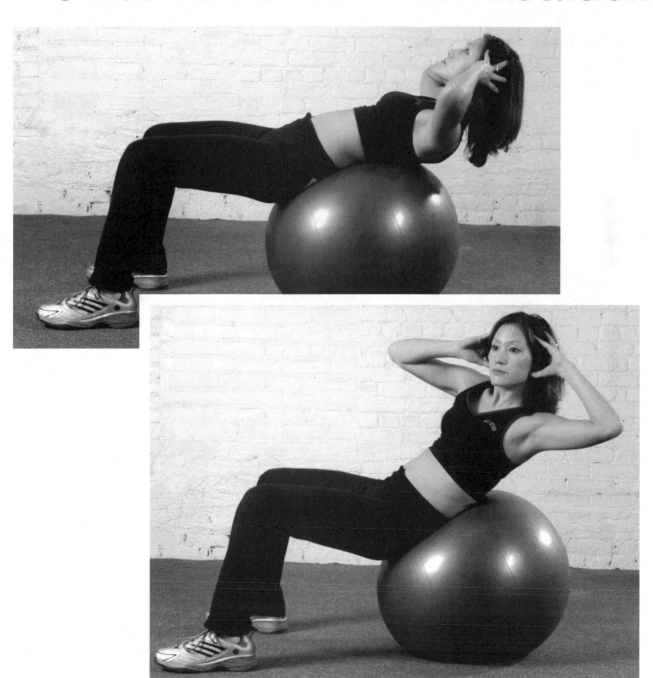

Swiss Ball Crunch...

This exercise requires incredible balance as well as strong abs. It may take you a while to get the form just right. But keep working at it. You'll be glad that you did!

TECHNIQUE AND FORM

1 Lie on a Swiss ball in the crunch position: feet flat on the floor, knees bent at about 90 degrees, and your back conformed to the ball.

2 With your belly button pulled toward your spine, crunch up diagonally by bringing your right armpit toward your left hip.

3 As you do so, simultaneously lift your left leg off the floor and bring it slightly toward your right shoulder.

4 When your left foot is 6 to 12 inches off the ground and your right shoulder blade is completely off the ball, hold that crunch position for a moment or two before slowly lowering yourself back to the ball and repeating on the other side.

5 Continue alternating for the desired number of reps.

TRAINER'S TIPS

✪ Avoid moving abruptly; smooth, controlled movements will help you maintain your balance.

✪ All the movement in this exercise should occur in the hip joint; do not bend and straighten the knee to bring the your leg up.

. . . with Cross Body Leg Lift

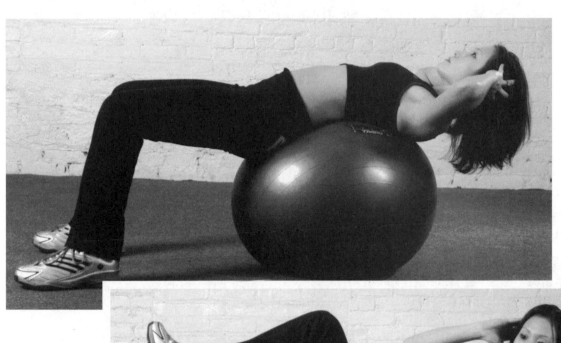

Swiss Ball Bridge

Wait until you try this one: Once you can knock out 30 seconds straight you'll have a seriously strong mid-section. Just don't celebrate your accomplishment with a hot-fudge sundae!

TECHNIQUE AND FORM

1 Kneel with a Swiss ball in front of you; place your forearms on the ball.

2 Lift your knees off the floor and straighten your legs so that only the balls of your feet are in contact with the floor. Your upper arms should be bent on top of the ball.

3 Make sure that your back is flat and your pelvis is in a neutral position by pulling your belly button to your spine, hollowing out your waist, and simultaneously tucking in your glutes.

4 Hold this position for 30 to 60 seconds while breathing through pursed lips.

5 Repeat for the desired number of reps.

TRAINER'S TIPS

◈ Don't allow your hips to sag toward the floor at any time during the exercise; doing so places strain on the lower back.

◈ Be aware of proper form: Don't hike your hips up into the air; keep your back straight. Your body should form a diagonal line from your feet to your head. Stay propped up on your forearms and keep your chest away from the ball.

Swiss Ball Bridge

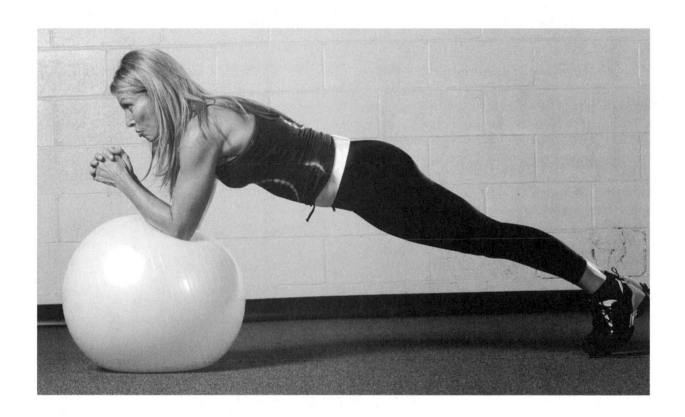

Swiss Ball Praying Mantis

This is another exercise in which looks can be deceiving. You may think it's going to be easy, but if you follow the form tips exactly, you should find it to be an extremely challenging exercise.

TECHNIQUE AND FORM

1 Kneel with a Swiss ball in front of you. Interlock your fingers and place your hands and lower forearms on the ball.

2 Allow the ball to roll forward slowly and let your torso and thighs move with it.

3 In the finish position your arms should be almost completely straight and your body forming a diagonal line from your knees to your head.

4 Hold this position for a moment or two before using your abdominal muscles to pull the ball back to the starting position.

5 Repeat for the desired number of reps.

TRAINER'S TIPS

Control the speed of the ball with your abs as it rolls away from you. Don't let it go too fast, or you're liable to take a spill.

Keep your belly button pulled to your spine throughout the movement to protect your back from potential strain.

Avoid trying to use your arms to pull the ball back in; let your abdominal muscles do the work.

Swiss Ball Praying Mantis

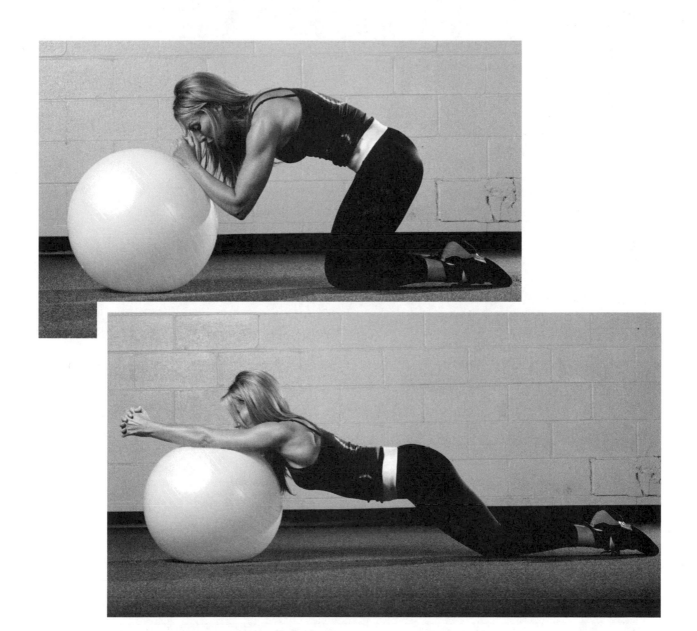

Chapter 6

Medicine Ball Exercises

6

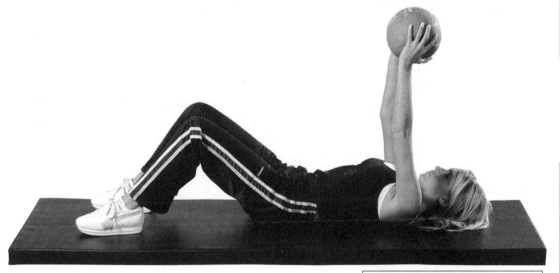

The great thing about working with medicine balls is that they allow you to train your abs for the types of explosive movements you perform during many common sport and leisure activities. Plus, since they're so affordable they offer an excellent alternative to expensive gym equipment.

THE BODY SCULPTING BIBLE FOR ABS

WOMEN'S EDITION

Medicine Ball Kneeling Throw

In this drill your abdominal muscles perform two jobs: (1) they help generate the power you need to throw the ball onto the floor; and (2) they help decelerate your torso so that your momentum doesn't force you forward onto the floor. You don't need a partner to do this exercise—but it's helpful to have someone fetch the ball for you!

TECHNIQUE AND FORM

1 Kneel on an exercise mat while holding an 8- to 12-pound medicine ball between your hands.

2 Extend your arms straight up overhead and pull your abs into your spine.

3 Keeping your arms straight, use your abdominals to quickly and forcefully throw the ball as hard as you can onto the floor about a foot or so in front of you.

4 You should finish the movement with your upper body almost parallel to the floor and your arms extended behind you.

5 Have a partner retrieve the ball for you or get it yourself and repeat the drill for the desired number of reps.

TRAINER'S TIPS

✪ Keep your arms as straight as possible and concentrate on using core power to throw the ball.

✪ Forcibly exhaling as you explode the ball into the floor can increase the intensity of the contraction.

✪ Throw the ball far enough away from you so that it doesn't bounce back up and hit you in the face but not so far as to reduce the effectiveness of the exercise.

Medicine Ball Kneeling Throw

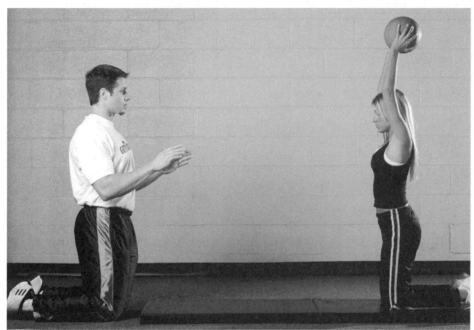

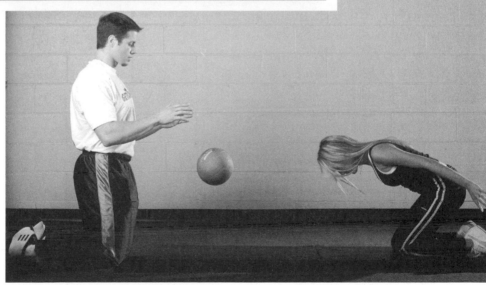

Medicine Ball Woodchopper

Just as with the Medicine Ball Kneeling Explosive Throw on the previous page, this exercise requires you to combine an explosive contraction with a rapid deceleration of the abdominals. That means it's important to stand firm and not allow your momentum to move your feet in the bottom position.

TECHNIQUE AND FORM

1 Stand with your feet shoulder width apart and your knees slightly bent.

2 Hold the medicine ball with your arms extended in front of you.

3 Lift your arms over your right shoulder as you pull your abs into your spine.

4 Quickly and forcefully "chop" the ball down in a sweeping diagonal motion across your body so that you end up with your torso flexed across your thighs and the ball just outside of your left calf. (Don't let go of the ball.)

5 Bring the ball back up in the same sweeping motion and repeat for the desired number of reps before switching to the other side.

TRAINER'S TIPS

⊗ Keep your arms as straight as possible and focus on sweeping the ball down across your body.

⊗ Avoid shortening the movement by bringing the ball only next to your upper thigh; be sure and get it down next to your calf.

Medicine Ball Woodchopper

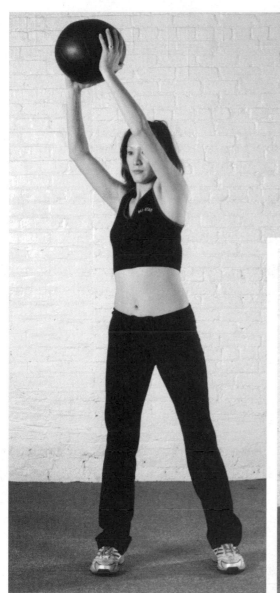

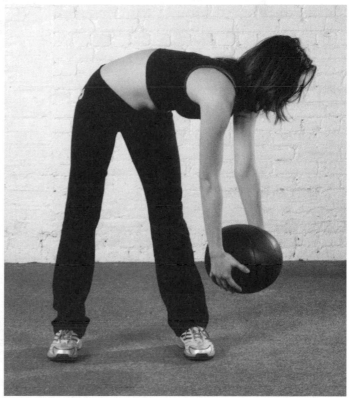

Medicine Ball Overhead Sit-Up

This is an extremely challenging exercise provided that you don't use momentum to propel your torso off of the floor. So remember: No cheating!

TECHNIQUE AND FORM

1 Lie on an exercise mat. Hold a 4- to 6-pound medicine ball in your hand with your arms extended over your head.

2 Keeping your arms straight and the ball directly over your head, sit up until your chest almost touches your thighs. Maintain proper sit-up posture.

3 Lower yourself back to the starting position.

4 Repeat for the desired number of reps.

TRAINER'S TIPS

❷ Avoid "throwing" your upper body forward to generate momentum. It completely destroys the training effect.

❷ Lower yourself slowly to take advantage of the negative portion of the movement.

❷ Once you become more advanced, you can use a heavier medicine ball.

Medicine Ball Overhead Sit-Up

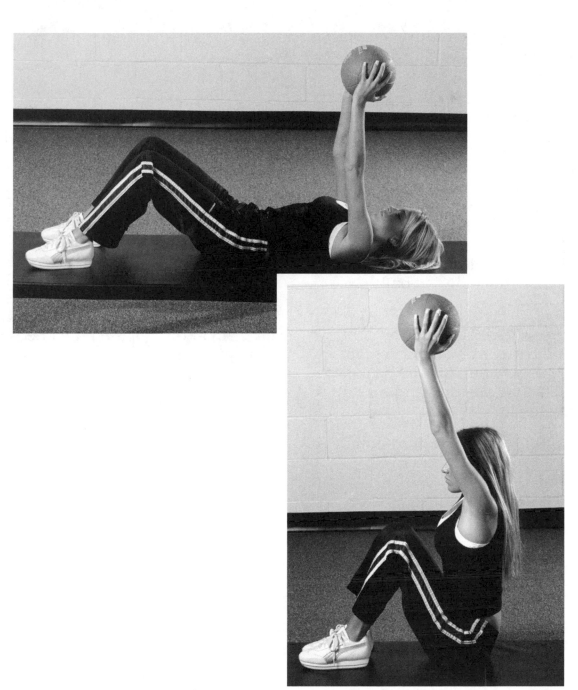

Medicine Ball Bicycle

This exercise takes a little coordination but the intense abdominal burn you get will be worth the time it takes to learn the moves.

TECHNIQUE AND FORM

❶ Lie on your back with your knees slightly bent and only your heels touching the floor.

❷ With your arms extended out to your sides and a 4- to 6-pound medicine ball in one hand, sit up as you simultaneously lift the leg opposite from the one holding the ball.

❸ As you bring that leg toward your chest, pass the ball under it to the opposite hand. As soon as you do, immediately lower yourself back down to the starting position and repeat on the other side.

❹ Continue for the desired number of reps.

TRAINER'S TIPS

✪ Keep your movement, passing the medicine ball from one hand to the other, as smooth and fluid as possible. Avoid resting in the bottom position.

✪ Try to lift both your lower and upper body at the same rate so they meet in the middle.

✪ Use your abs to bring your chest toward your thigh and vice versa. Do not bend and straighten the knees to bring your legs in.

Medicine Ball Bicycle

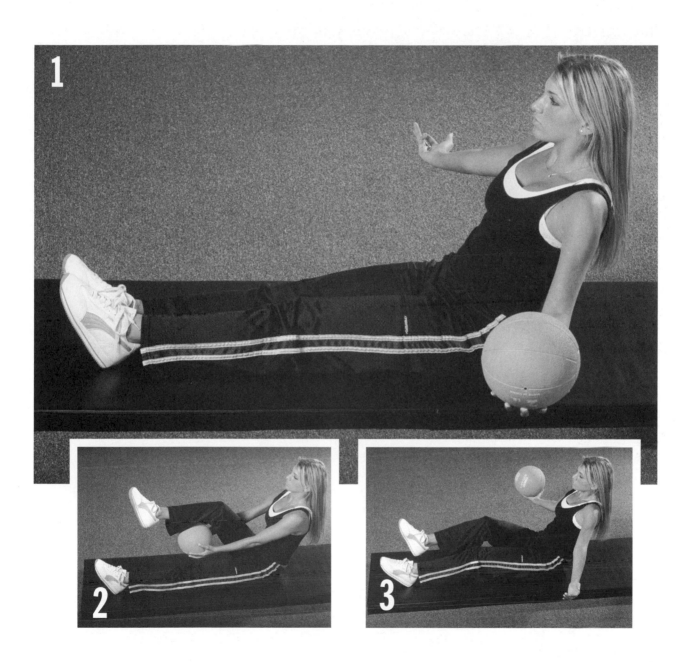

Chapter 7

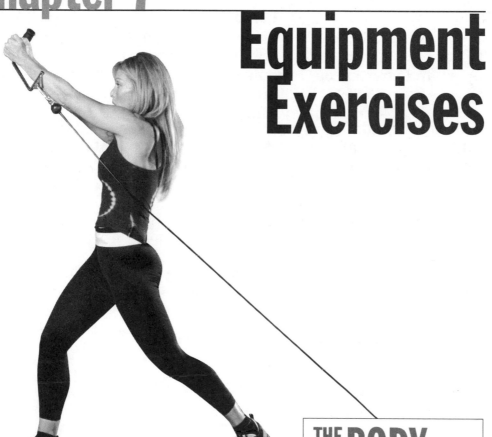

Equipment Exercises

7

Besides Swiss Balls and medicine balls there are lots of other tools you can use to give your abs a great workout. From the inexpensive (like dumbbells) to the more elaborate (like cable stations), they can all provide a terrific workout.

THE **BODY SCULPTING BIBLE** FOR **ABS**

High-to-Low Cable Woodchopper

An excellent exercise for developing rotational power, the Woodchopper will have your abs and obliques begging for mercy. Show them who's boss!

TECHNIQUE AND FORM

1 Stand sideways in the middle of a cable station with your feet about shoulder width apart and your knees slightly bent.

2 Reach up and over your right shoulder with both arms and grab hold of the handle attached to the high pulley.

3 Keeping your arms straight and knees slightly bent, bring the weight down in a sweeping, diagonal motion across your body until the cable handle ends up outside your left calf and your torso is flexed across your legs.

4 Slowly reverse direction, returning the weight to the starting position.

5 Repeat for the desired number of reps before switching to the other side.

TRAINER'S TIPS

Keep your arms straight and focus on using your core to pull the weight down and across your body. Avoid pulling the weight with just your arms.

Stand firm; try not to move or reposition your feet during the exercise. Stand (and stay) in a ready, athletic stance with your feet apart and knees bent. Generate power with your core, not your legs.

Exhale as you bring the weight down to intensify the contraction.

High-to-Low Cable Woodchopper

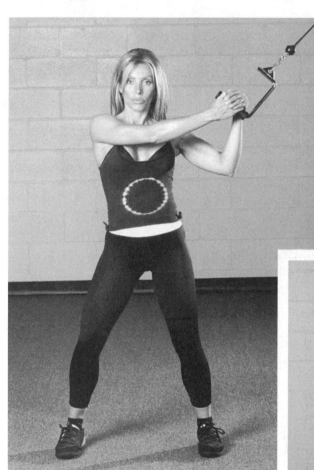

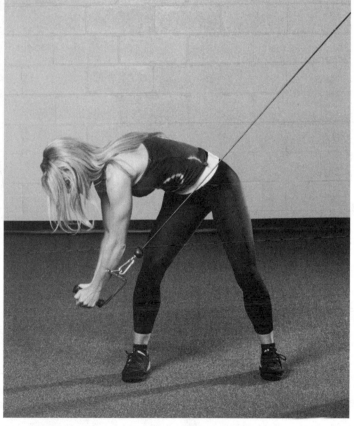

Low-to-High Cable Woodchopper

This Woodchopper is guaranteed to please the toddlers in your life who like to be picked up. Just make sure you strengthen your abs so you can lift them as often as they ask.

TECHNIQUE AND FORM

1 Begin in the same position as for the High-to-Low Woodchopper on the previous page, only this time grab the right *lower* pulley attachment with both of your hands. Your arms should be straight and your hands positioned just outside your right hip.

2 Keep your shoulders and hips squared and facing forward as you work the weight upward in a sweeping diagonal movement.

3 Once the weight is high over your left shoulder, pause for a moment or two and then lower the weight back to the starting position.

4 Repeat for the desired number of reps.

TRAINER'S TIPS

✪ Just as you did for the High-to-Low Woodchopper, keep your arms straight throughout the exercise.

✪ Grab the pulley using a hand-over-hand grip. Keep the hand of the side you're going to on the bottom. This helps reduce the tendency to pull the weight with your opposite arm and increases the demand on your core.

✪ Stand firm; try not to shift or move your feet as you perform the exercise.

Low-to-High Cable Woodchopper

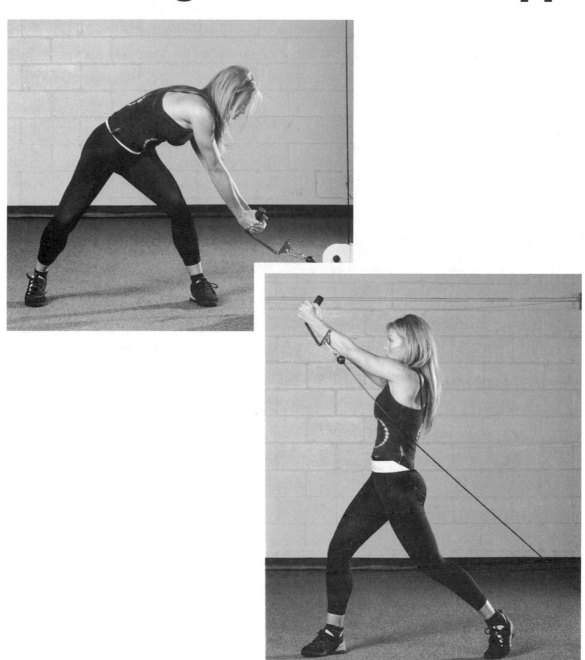

Cable Crunch

This is one of those exercises that for some reason or other people tend to perform incorrectly. Make sure you go over directions very carefully before you start.

TECHNIQUE AND FORM

❶ Grab the high pulley attachment of the cable station with both hands and kneel about two feet from and facing the weight stack.

❷ Keeping your elbows slightly bent, tuck your head between your arms and crunch your rib cage toward your pelvis.

❸ When your elbows are just about touch the middle of your thighs, slowly uncoil your spine and return to the starting position.

❹ Repeat for the desired number of reps.

TRAINER'S TIPS

✪ Flexing your spine is the key to this exercise. To do it correctly, imagine someone holding a broomstick horizontally in front of you about 6 inches away from your belly button. When crunching, bring your elbows down and over the stick without touching it.

✪ Keep the same degree of bend in your elbows throughout the exercise; don't bend them any more or straighten them.

✪ Keep your hips in a fixed position with your rear end off your heels. Don't let them move up and down.

Cable Crunch

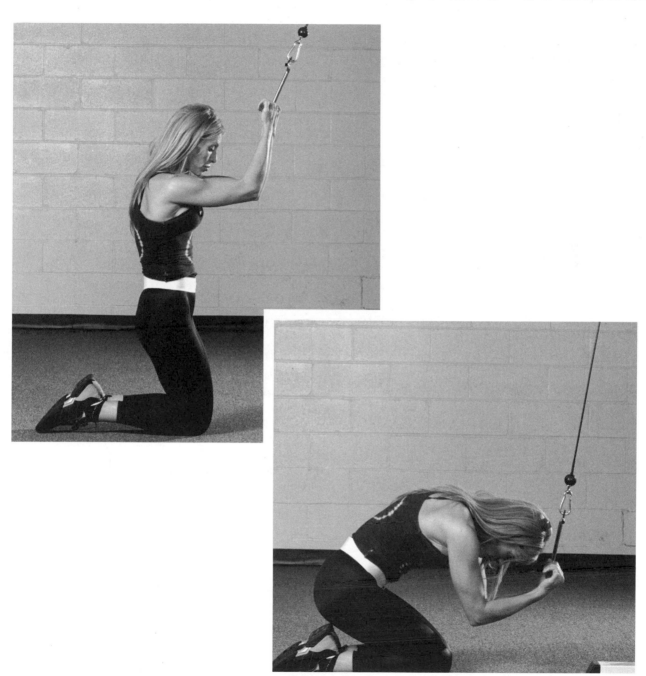

Saxon Side Bends

A word of warning, these are *much* harder than the classic side bend, in which you hold a dumbbell at arm's length next to your thigh. Use caution.

TECHNIQUE AND FORM

1 Grab a pair of light (3- to 5-pound) dumbbells and stand with your feet shoulder width apart and knees slightly bent.

2 Straighten your arms over your head so that the weights line up directly over your shoulders.

3 Pulling your abs to your spine, slowly lean your upper body as far to one side as you can without feeling pain.

4 Once you're leaning over as far as you can, use your abs and obliques to pull yourself back up to the center.

5 Repeat on the other side and then continue for the desired number reps.

TRAINER'S TIPS

⊘ The most common error you can make is rotating your torso as you lean. Keep the movement lateral by making sure your shoulders and hips face forward at all times—no twisting.

⊘ Avoid locking your knees (keep them soft), arching your back (maintain neutral spine), or bending and straightening your arms (keep them straight).

⊘ You can use a medicine ball in place of weights for this exercise. Hold one ball with both hands as you do the exercise.

Saxon Side Bends

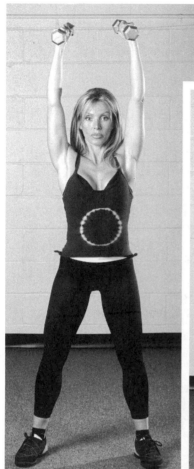
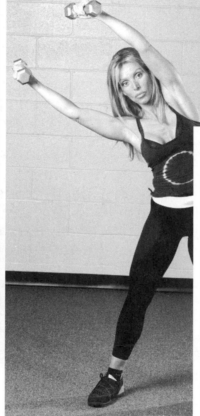
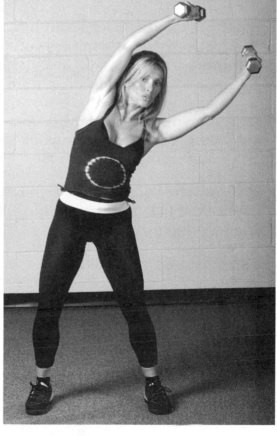

Slant Board Reverse Crunch

When you do this exercise, imagine folding your body in half at the waist; avoid just bending and straightening your legs.

TECHNIQUE AND FORM

1 Lie on an abdominal slant board or decline weight bench with your arms extended above your head. Hold the back of the bench for support.

2 Lift your legs so that your knees are above your hips and your legs form a 90-degree angle.

3 Slowly lift your legs and hips toward your chest, making sure to round your lower back and lift your tailbone off the bench as you do so. When you are in the contracted position your thighs should be almost touching your chest with your lower back rounded.

4 Hold that position for a moment or two before lowering yourself back to the starting position.

5 Repeat for the desired number of reps.

TRAINER'S TIPS

◆ The key in this exercise—as in many of the others—is spinal flexion. Pulling your legs in just by bending your knees will do little for your abs. Think of your pelvis as a bowl of water that you're dumping out onto your chest to get a feel for how to flex your spine.

◆ The difficulty of this exercise depends on the steepness of the incline. The steeper the incline, the more you have to overcome the effects of gravity.

◆ Don't lift your back too high off the bench. Lifting your lower back slightly should give you all the spinal flexion you need.

Slant Board Reverse Crunch

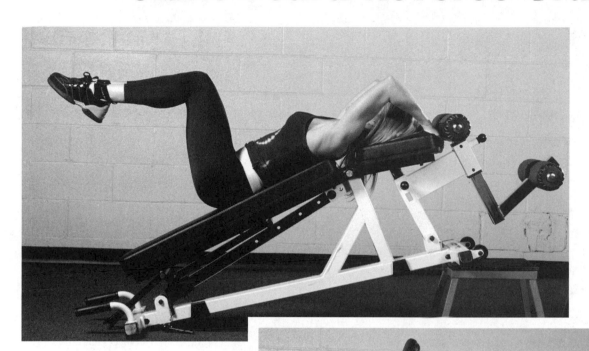

Hanging Leg Raises

This is probably the number one ab exercise that is most often performed incorrectly. That's because most people lack the strength to do the exercise the right way. But keep at it and you'll succeed.

TECHNIQUE AND FORM

1 Place your upper arms in a pair of Ab-Originals™ and hang from an overhead bar.

2 Without swinging, use your abs and hip flexors to pull your legs up and in toward your chest. As you do so, round your back and pull your thighs in as close to your chest as possible.

3 Exhale at the top of the motion and then slowly lower your legs to the starting position.

4 Repeat for the desired number of reps.

TRAINER'S TIPS

● Ab-Originals™ is a piece of equipment that almost any gym will own. If your gym doesn't own a set, suggest that it order them.

● Avoid swinging to start the momentum to lift your legs.

● Spinal flexion is key here. That means you have to lift your legs high enough so that your hips "roll" under your body slightly and your back rounds.

● Keeping your back straight and lifting only your knees places far too much emphasis on the hip flexors and works your abdominals only minimally.

● Lower your legs to the bottom position only to the point at which you can maintain a neutral pelvis. This will help keep tension on your abs and off of your lower back.

Hanging Leg Raises

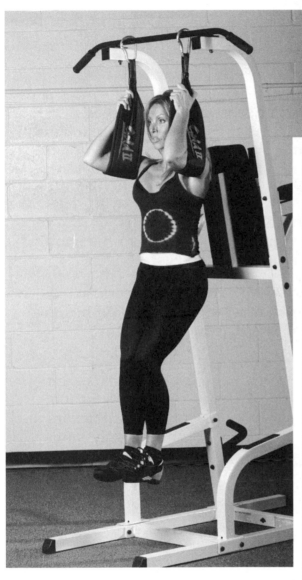

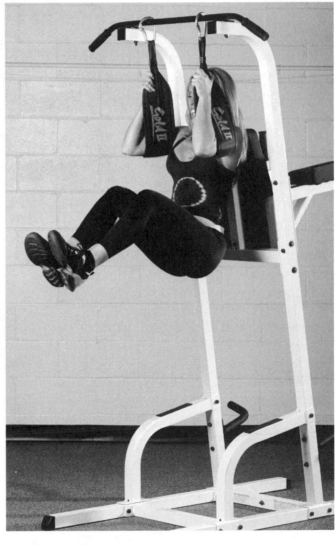

Hanging Oblique Raise

If you thought the Hanging Leg Raises were challenging, just wait until you get a load of this ab-blaster! Hang in there!

TECHNIQUE AND FORM

1 Start by positioning yourself in the Ab-Originals™ as though you were going to perform the Hanging Leg Raises on the previous page.

2 This time, however, keep your back straight as you lift your knees until your upper thighs are parallel to the floor.

3 Holding that position, use your obliques to slowly lift your right hip toward your right armpit.

4 Once you get as high as you can go, pause for a moment or two before lowering yourself back to the original position and then proceed to the other side.

5 Repeat for the desired number of reps.

TRAINER'S TIPS

✪ Concentrate on using your obliques to pull your hip up toward your armpits.

✪ Keep your knees bent as you lower yourself; don't let your legs straighten between reps. Only after completing a full set of reps should you lower your legs.

✪ When you're in the contracted position, your shins should be diagonal to the floor.

Hanging Oblique Raise

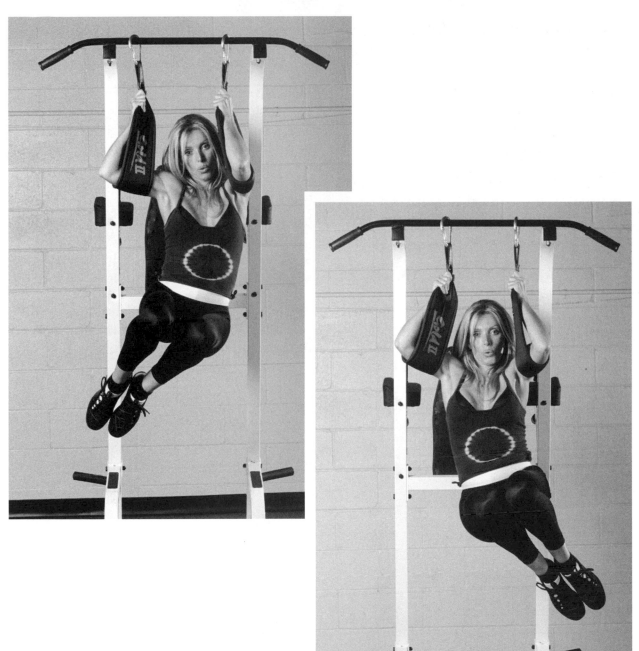

High Chair Scissors

This exercise offers an interesting little twist on one of the more ho-hum ab exercises.

TECHNIQUE AND FORM

1 Get into an abdominal high chair by propping yourself up on your elbows and forearms.

2 Allowing your legs to hang beneath you with a slight bend in your knees, lift the right leg toward your chest. Leaving the left leg hanging.

3 Slowly lower the right leg while simultaneously lifting the right leg, and so on.

4 Repeat for the desired number of reps.

TRAINER'S TIPS

◆ Initiate the leg movement at your hip joint; don't bend and straighten your knees; it's tough, but stay with it!

◆ To reduce the possibility of lower back strain or injury, keep your lower back pressed flat against the chair's pad and your feet hanging down slightly in front of you, where you can see them in the starting position

◆ Try to achieve spinal flexion by lifting your lower back slightly off of the pad in the contracted position.

◆ Avoid letting the hanging leg pull up as you lift the working leg; it should remain as straight as possible.

High Chair Scissors

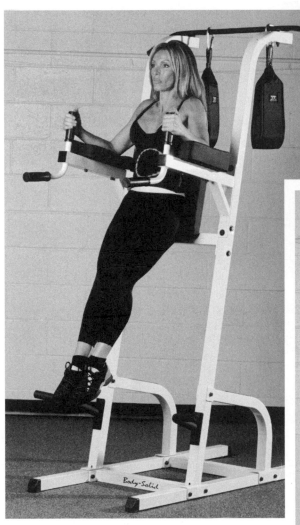

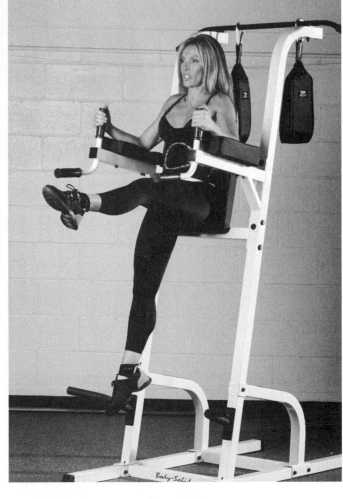

Chapter 6
Lower Back Exercises

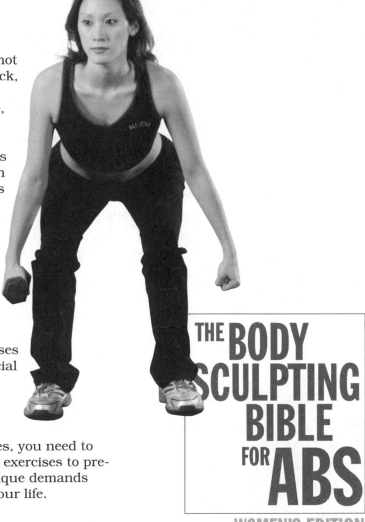

The following exercises not only train your lower back, but they also work your entire core. For example, the Overhead Squat, although it involves no quick movements, places an incredible demand on your lower back muscles to help stabilize your position. Not to mention the amount of work your abs are forced to do to stabilize the bar. It is this ability to force your abs and lower back to work together as a unit that makes these exercises so tremendously beneficial from a practical standpoint. Since you will rarely, if ever, isolate your abs or lower back during everyday activities, you need to include some integrated exercises to prepare yourself for the unique demands imposed by just living your life.

6

THE BODY SCULPTING BIBLE FOR ABS

WOMEN'S EDITION

Supermans

If you work your abs, you must work your lower back. Here's a simple but effective exercise to target those often-ignored spinal erectors. (If you don't like to think of yourself as Superman, imagine being Wonder Woman!)

TECHNIQUE AND FORM

1 Lie flat on your stomach with your arms extended straight out in front of you and your legs extended straight out behind you.

2 Keeping your arms and legs perfectly straight, simultaneously lift your arms, chest, and legs a few inches off the floor.

3 Once there, hold the position for a second or two before lowering again.

4 Repeat for the desired number of reps.

TRAINER'S TIPS

◈ Make sure that you lift yourself off of the mat in a slow, controlled manner; avoid jerking yourself up into position.

◈ Try to look at the floor throughout the movement to avoid unnecessary hyperextension of the neck.

◈ For a useful variation of this exercise, begin in the same starting position as described in Step 1. Next, lift your right arm and left leg off the floor at the same time. Switch arms/legs and repeat. You can even perform this variation on all fours, lifting and extending your left arm and your right leg and vice versa.

Supermans

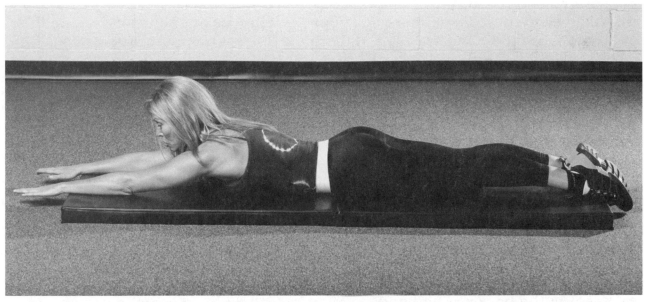

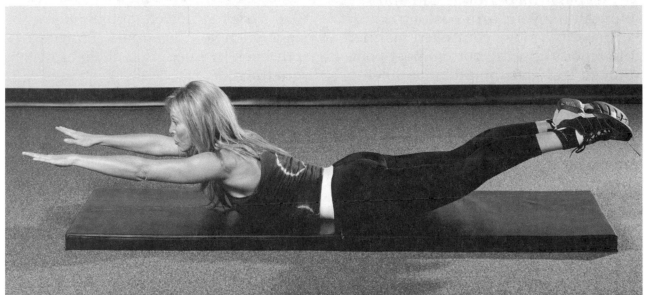

Overhead Squats

You may need to work on improving your flexibility before you can execute this movement properly; but stay with it, because this is an important exercise.

TECHNIQUE AND FORM

1 Hold a barbell with your palms facing down. Your hands should be approximately twice your shoulder width apart.

2 With your feet about shoulder width apart and your knees slightly bent, press the bar up overhead until your arms are completely straight.

3 Keeping the bar overhead and maintaining your arm position, lower yourself in a slow, controlled manner into a squat. In the bottommost position your thighs should be parallel to the floor.

4 Once there, pause momentarily before bringing the weight back up to the starting position.

5 Repeat for the desired number of reps.

TRAINER'S TIPS

✪ Make sure that your arms are as straight as possible throughout the lift and stay just beyond your peripheral vision. Allowing your arms to drift forward can increase strain on the upper and lower back.

✪ Keep your abs pulled to your spine throughout the lift and especially in the bottom position.

✪ It's easy to neglect spinal alignment when you do squats. Protect your back by keeping it straight while squatting.

Overhead Squats

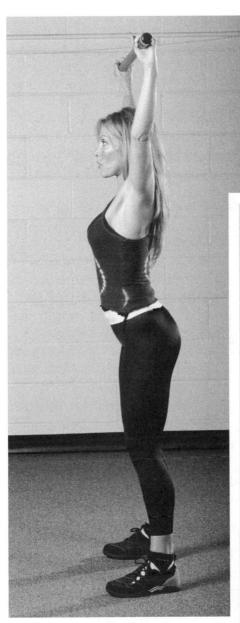

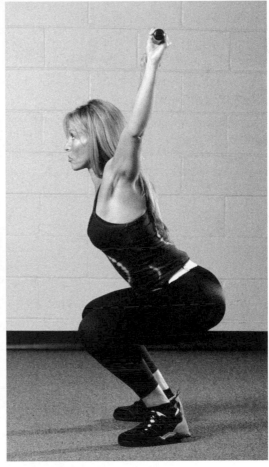

Good Mornings

This is a very advanced exercise—but when done correctly a terrific one—so please use caution. You need to fully concentrate on your form as you do the exercise to get the full benefit and reduce the risk of injury.

TECHNIQUE AND FORM

1 Place a barbell across your upper back so that it rests on your upper trapezius, just above your shoulder blades.

2 With your feet about shoulder width apart and knees slightly bent, lean forward, breaking at the hips, until your torso is just about parallel to the ground. Pause momentarily before bringing the bar back up to the starting position.

3 Repeat for the desired number of reps.

TRAINER'S TIPS

⊗ Concentrate during every rep for this exercise because losing your alignment can lead to injury.

⊗ Keep your shoulder blades together and your chest out throughout the exercise.

⊗ Don't alter the amount of bend in your knees as you raise and lower the weight. Start with a slight bend in your knees and concentrate on using the hips as the fulcrum of the movement.

⊗ It is crucial that you maintain an arch in your lower back as you lower and raise the weight. Allowing your back to round when your spine is flexed forward greatly increases your risk of injury.

⊗ Concentrate on driving your heels into the floor to lift the weight back up. Do not try and simply extend your spine.

Good Mornings

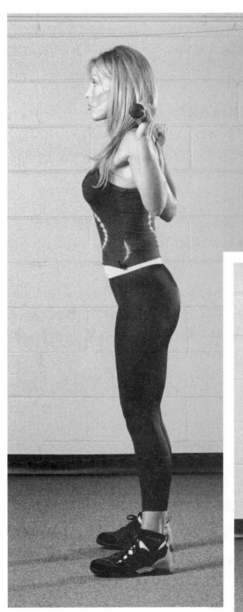

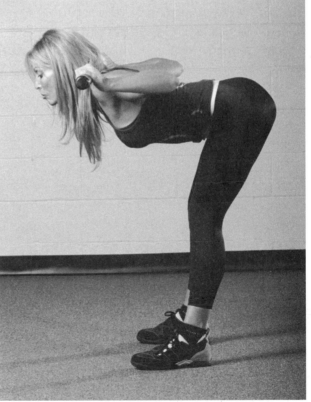

Suitcase Dead Lifts

The Suitcase Dead Lift is aptly titled, but it can be a bit awkward to perform, so you need to start slowly and with a light dumbbell. The key to the exercise is to lift the weight as if both sides of your body were equally loaded.

TECHNIQUE AND FORM

1 Hold a light dumbbell as if you were picking up a suitcase. Stand with your feet shoulder width apart and knees slightly bent.

2 Slowly squat with the weight, keeping your torso as erect as possible.

3 Once you've descended to the point where your thighs are parallel to the floor, pause momentarily before pressing back up to the starting position. Repeat for the desired number of reps before moving the barbell to the opposite hand.

TRAINER'S TIPS

Keep your shoulders and hips squared forward; do not allow the arm holding the dumbbell to pull your body into a lopsided posture.

Keep you abs pulled to your spine and maintain a slight arch in your lower back throughout the exercise.

If you're a beginner, you can even start this exercise using a broomstick in place of a dumbbell just to get a feel for what's required.

Suitcase Dead Lifts

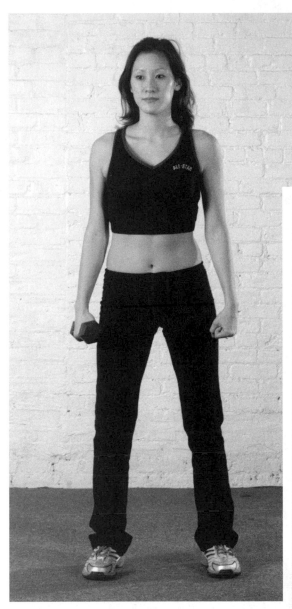

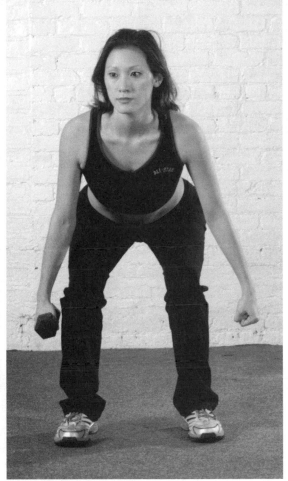

Unilateral Romanian Dead Lift

This one's almost as difficult to perform as it is awkward to say. Once you get it down however, you can just feel that it's doing your body some good.

TECHNIQUE AND FORM

1 Stand with your feet about shoulder width apart and knees slightly bent.

2 Keeping your torso straight and tall, lift one foot an inch or two off of the floor.

3 Once you feel balanced, maintain a slight bend in the other knee as you slowly lean forward by sticking your hips back and bringing your torso over toward the floor. As you descend, be sure to maintain the arch in your lower back.

4 Once your torso is just about parallel to the floor, pause momentarily before lifting back up into the starting position.

TRAINER'S TIPS

Keep the non-working leg about an inch or two from the floor throughout the exercise. Avoid allowing it to lean against the other leg for support.

Maintain a slight arch in your back throughout the exercise.

Do not allow your back to round at any point during the lift.

If you're just starting out, try the exercise with a weight: Allow your arms to hang straight down beneath your shoulders. Once you've mastered the lift with just your body weight, perform the exercise with some light dumbbells in your hands.

Unilateral Romanian Dead Lift

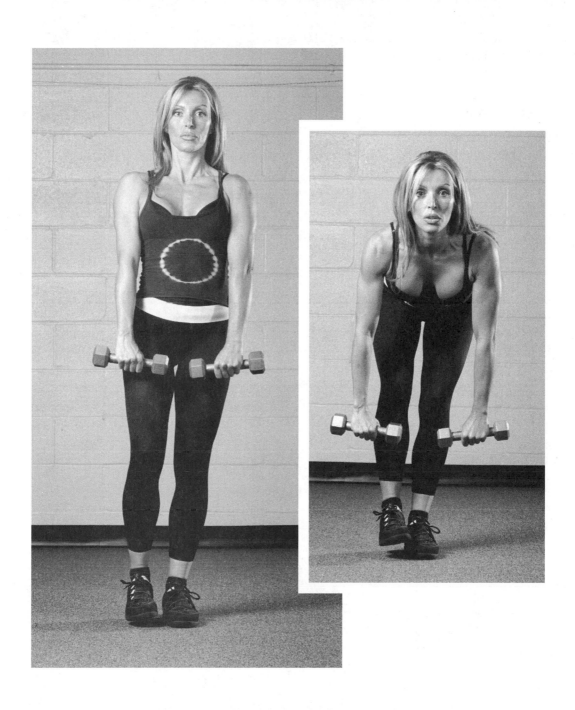

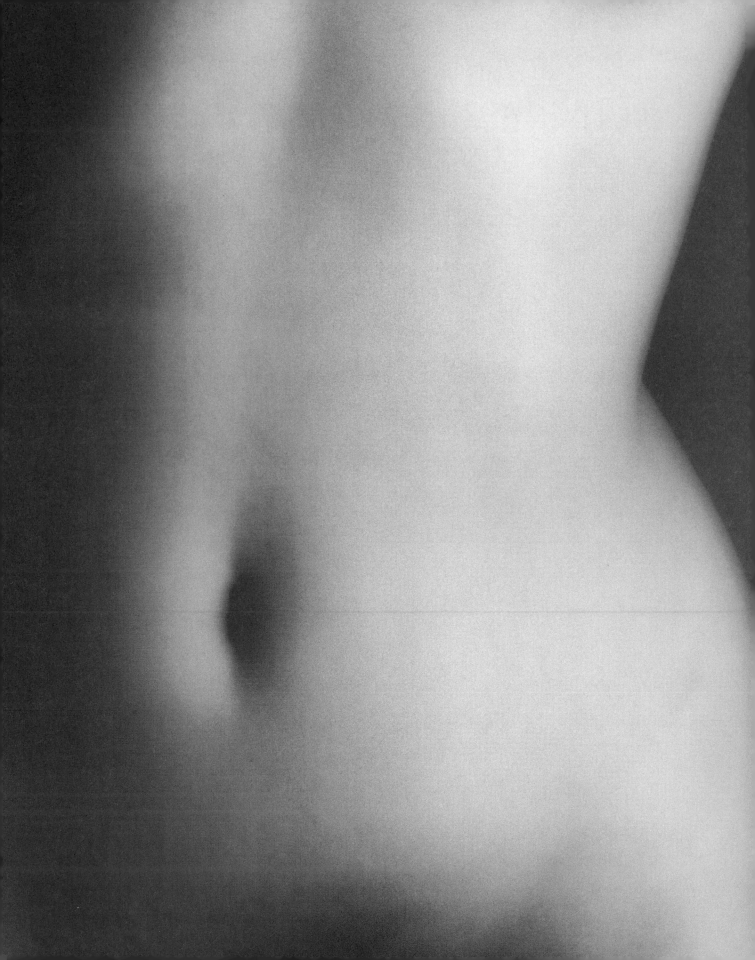

Part 3

THE BODY SCULPTING BIBLE FOR ABS 14-DAY WORKOUTS

THE **BODY SCULPTING BIBLE** FOR **ABS**

WOMEN'S EDITION

Chapter 9
The Workouts

Whether you're just starting out or are already on the road to abs-to-die-for, there's a workout here for you. We've even included an Ab Workout To Go that you can do anytime, anywhere!

9

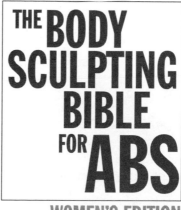

GETTING STARTED

You want a sleek, sexy waistline? You've come to the right place. It won't happen overnight; in fact, it'll take work, dedication, consistency, and intensity on your part. But with our 14-Day Ab Sculpting Workouts, you'll be off to a good start.

All of our workouts were designed to be as user friendly as possible. We've set them in chart format, so that you can Xerox the pages and take them to the gym with you.

We've also included the page numbers of the exercises in the chart to make it easy to refer back to the photographs and descriptions.

First things first. If you haven't been doing much—or any—ab work lately, you'll want to start your program with the 14-Day Break-In Workouts. They were designed to get your midsection up and running, so to speak; to ready you for the more intense work to come.

Already in pretty good shape? Go ahead and start with the 14-Day Ab Sculpting Workouts. These more advanced programs will get your core into the best shape of your life.

SCHEDULING YOUR AB WORKOUTS

When should you do your ab training? If your abs are your priority, do these workouts prior to or on a separate day from any strength training you do. Otherwise, you can do ab work right after your strength work—although as the intensity level of the exercises increases, you may find that more difficult to do as the weeks progress.

THE BREAK-IN WORKOUTS

Here's what you can expect from the 14-Day Break-In Workouts:

You'll do abs workouts on three (non-consecutive) days a week for at least two weeks.

If you haven't already, you should start incorporating two to three total-body strength workouts into your schedule as well as two to three days of interval cardio work.

Start each of your workouts with an overall total-body warm-up and then progress to the specific warm-ups on pages 24 to 39.

If, after two weeks, you don't feel ready to move on, don't. Just repeat the 14-Day Break-In Workouts for another several weeks or until you feel ready to proceed. Remember, the only person you're competing with is your old, out-of-shape self.

THE 14-DAY ABS SCULPTING WORKOUTS

Here's the low-down on these workouts:

There are two workouts, Level I and Level II. Each workout is comprised of a six-week program that has been broken down into 14-day segments. That means during each level you'll do six weeks of abs work, changing the specific workouts every two weeks.

The workouts have been designed to be progressive, becoming more difficult as the week progress. That means you need to do them in order—Level I first and then Level II—with no skipping around.

By the end of the first six weeks, you should be feeling and seeing significant results *as long as you've also been following a sound diet and incorporating interval cardio work into your life.*

Level II is an advanced workout. (That does not mean the Level I exercises are "easy," as you will discover!) So if you're not able to perform the exercises with proper form—and proper form is of paramount importance—repeat the previous 14-day workout.

You'll notice that as the weeks progress you're actually doing fewer reps. What's up? As the number of reps decrease you'll need to

THE ZONE-TONE METHOD

The mind-to-muscle connection, coupled with proper exercise technique and form, are crucial if you want to stimulate the necessary muscle fibers needed to create dynamite abs. That may sound like common sense, but most people neglect the mental aspect of training. How about you? When you're getting ready to do an exercise, do you ever stop to think about exactly what muscles you're about to train? Well, you should, because it really will increase the effectiveness of any exercise you do. I've designed a technique, called the Zone-Tone Method, that will help you do just that.

The Zone-Tone method helps you to mentally focus on and preisolate specific muscles just before and during an exercise. The technique is easy to grasp and will deliver enormous benefits to your fitness program. Combining proper form and technique with the Zone-Tone method will help you reach your goals more quickly.

There are only two simple steps to the Zone-Tone method:

❶ Zone in on the individual muscles you intend to train before you begin the exercise. Before each set, before each rep, concentrate on the individual muscles you'll be working. Now tense and flex that muscle as hard as comfortably possible before performing the exercise. What you're doing is preparing the muscle by isolating it even before the exercise begins. This is making the mind-to-muscle connection.

❷ Maintain your mind-to-muscle connection during the exercise. Feel the muscle elongate (stretch) and contract and flex the muscle as hard as you can as you did in Step 1 (except now you flex during the exercise). This is crucial; there's no point in activating the muscles before the exercise begins if you don't do it during the exercise, too.

Most people waste their time by exercising without thinking about what they're doing. That's fine if you're content with average results, but who wants to be average? On the other hand, if you want to compound your efforts exponentially, then you must effectively develop the mind-to-muscle connection. I guarantee that if you use this Zone-Tone technique with the 14-Day Ab Sculpting Workout, you'll achieve better results in less time.

add resistance. That could mean, for example, using a heavier medicine ball for the Woodchoppers, holding a plate on your chest as you do the Slow Sit-Ups, or wearing ankle weights and holding light dumbbells while you do the Supermans. In every instance, the weight needs to be heavy enough that you can just complete the given number of reps, but not so heavy that it screws up your form.

One last thing. Before you get started, you should review the principles of my Zone-Tone training technique, which I laid out in *The Body Sculpting Bible for Women*. There's a short refresher above.

Wake Up Your Abs Daily Workout

SPECIAL INSTRUCTIONS FOR DAILY WORKOUTS

- Warm up and then immediately begin exercises.
- Perform all exercises with the designated amount of rest between every exercise.
- For any exercise that requires weight, use one heavy enough so that you can just complete the required number of reps with good form.
- Swap in the Power Workout once or twice a week to intensify your workout.

DAY 1			MONDAY
No.	Warm-Up	Page No.	Reps/Time
1	Alternating Knee to Chest	24	10 on each side
2	The Roll	26	10
3	Pelvic Tilt	28	10
4	Press Up	30	10
5	Rotational Stretch	32	8 on each side
No.	Exercise	Page No.	Reps/Time
1	Towel Crunch	42	20
2	Knee-In	52	10
3	Lateral Bridge	48	10 on each side
4	Supermans	118	20

10 second rest between exercises

DAY 2			TUESDAY
No.	Warm-Up	Page No.	Reps/Time
1	Alternating Knee to Chest	24	10 on each side
2	The Roll	26	10
3	Press Up	30	10
No.	Exercise	Page No.	Reps/Time
1	Bicycle	58	10 on each side
2	Swiss Ball Crunch	64	20
3	Crunch with Lateral Flexion	44	10 on each side

5 second rest between exercises

DAY 3			WEDNESDAY
No.	**Warm-Up**	**Page No.**	**Reps/Time**
1	Alternating Knee to Chest	24	10 on each side
2	The Roll	26	10
3	Press Up	30	10
No.	**Exercise**	**Page No.**	**Reps/Time**
1	Towel Crunch with Weight	42	10
2	Swiss Ball Oblique Crunch	66	10 on each side
3	Windshield Wipers	54	10 on each side

20 second rest between exercises

DAY 4			THURSDAY
No.	**Warm-Up**	**Page No.**	**Reps/Time**
1	Alternating Knee to Chest	24	10 on each side
2	The Roll	26	10
3	Press Up	30	10
No.	**Exercise**	**Page No.**	**Reps/Time**
1	Slow Sit-Up	46	8
2	Swiss Ball Crunch with Rotation	80	10 on each side
3	Swiss Ball Bridge	84	30–60 second hold

10 second rest between exercises

DAY 5			FRIDAY
No.	**Warm-Up**	**Page No.**	**Reps/Time**
1	Alternating Knee to Chest	24	10 on each side
2	The Roll	26	10
3	Pelvic Tilt	28	10
4	Press Up	30	10
5	Rotational Stretch	32	8 on each side
No.	**Exercise**	**Page No.**	**Reps/Time**
1	V-Up	50	8
2	Swiss Ball Crunch with Weight	64	10
3	Twisting Pulse Up	56	10 on each side
4	Supermans	118	20

15 second rest between exercises

Power Workout

SPECIAL INSTRUCTIONS FOR POWER WORKOUT

- Warm up and then immediately begin exercises.
- Perform all exercises with only 5 seconds of rest in between.
- Rest for one minute after all exercises have been performed consecutively.
- Perform an Isometric Abdominal Contraction for 15 Seconds at the end of the set, then repeat.

No.	Warm-Up	Page No.	Reps/Time
POWER WORKOUT			

No.	Warm-Up	Page No.	Reps/Time
1	Alternating Knee to Chest	24	10 on each side
2	The Roll	26	10
3	Pelvic Tilt	28	10
4	Press Up	30	10
5	Rotational Stretch	32	8 on each side
No.	Exercise	Page No.	Reps/Time
1	Towel Crunch	42	20
2	Crunch with Lateral Flexion	44	10
3	V-Up	50	8
4	Slow Sit-Up	46	8
5	Lateral Bridge	48	10 on each side
6	Knee-In	52	10
7	Windshield Wipers	54	10 on each side
8	Twisting Pulse Up	56	10 on each side
9	Bicycles	58	10 on each side
10	Swiss Ball Crunch	64	20
11	Swiss Ball Oblique Crunch	66	10 on each side
12	Swiss Ball Crunch with Rotation	80	10 on each side
13	Swiss Ball Bridge	84	30 second hold

Break-In Workout: Week 1

- Perform three ab workouts each week.
- Begin to incorporate two to three total-body strength workouts and two to three days of interval cardio in your program.
- Start with a general warm-up and then proceed to the Ab Warm-Ups (pages 24 to 39) before beginning these workouts.

DAY 1

No.	Exercise	Page No.	Reps/Time
1	Bicycles	58	10 to 12
2	Slow Sit-Up	46	8 to 12
3	Saxon Side Bends	106	6 to 8 on each side
4	Swiss Ball Cobra	76	10 to 12

Perform as a circuit (one exercise after the other).

DAY 2

No.	Exercise	Page No.	Reps/Time
1	High Chair Scissors	114	6 to 8 on each side
2	Swiss Ball Bridge	84	20 to 30 seconds
3	Crunch with Lateral Flexion	44	8 to 10 on each side
4	Supermans	118	12 to 15

Perform as a circuit (one exercise after the other).

DAY 3

No.	Exercise	Page No.	Reps/Time
1	Bicycles	58	10 to 12
2	Slow Sit-Up	46	8 to 12
3	Saxon Side Bends	106	6 to 8 on each side
4	Swiss Ball Cobra	76	10 to 12

Perform as a circuit (one exercise after the other).

Break-In Workout: Week 2

SPECIAL INSTRUCTIONS FOR WEEKS 1 & 2

- Perform three ab workouts each week.
- Begin to incorporate two to three total-body strength workouts and two to three days of interval cardio in your program.
- Start with a general warm-up and then proceed to the Ab Warm-Ups (pages 26 to 43) before beginning these workouts.

DAY 1

No.	Exercise	Page No.	Reps/Time
1	High Chair Scissors	114	6 to 8 on each side
2	Swiss Ball Bridge	84	20 to 30 seconds
3	Crunch with Lateral Flexion	44	8 to 10 on each side
4	Supermans	118	12 to 15

Perform as a circuit (one exercise after the other).

DAY 2

No.	Exercise	Page No.	Reps/Time
1	Bicycles	58	10 to 12
2	Slow Sit-Up	46	8 to 12
3	Saxon Side Bends	106	6 to 8 on each side
4	Swiss Ball Cobra	76	10 to 12

Perform as a circuit (one exercise after the other).

DAY 3

No.	Exercise	Page No.	Reps/Time
1	High Chair Scissors	114	6 to 8 on each side
2	Swiss Ball Bridge	84	20 to 30 seconds
3	Crunch with Lateral Flexion	44	8 to 10 on each side
4	Supermans	118	12 to 15

Perform as a circuit (one exercise after the other).

14-Day Ab Sculpting Workout #1: Weeks 1 & 2

SPECIAL INSTRUCTIONS FOR WEEKS 1 & 2

- Perform three ab workouts each week. Incorporate two to three total-body strength workouts and two to three days of interval cardio in your program.
- Start with a general warm-up and then proceed to the Ab Warm-Ups (pages 24 to 39) before beginning these workouts.
- For any exercise that requires weight, use one heavy enough so that you can just complete the required number of reps with good form.

No.	Exercise	Page No.	Reps/Time
DAY 1			**FOCUS: CORE STABILITY**
1	Slow Sit-Up	46	10 to 12
2	Swiss Ball Bridge	84	30 to 60 seconds
3	Medicine Ball Woodchopper	92	10 to 12
4	Swiss Ball Cobra	76	10 to 12

Perform exercises as a circuit (one exercise after the other); rest 1 minute and then repeat entire circuit once or twice.

No.	Exercise	Page No.	Reps/Time
DAY 2			**FOCUS: CORE STRENGTH**
1	Slant Board Reverse Crunch	108	10 to 12
2	High-to-Low Cable Woodchopper	100	8 to 10 on each side
3	Knee-In	52	10 to 12
4	Suitcase Dead Lifts	124	8 to 10 on each side

Perform exercises as a circuit (one exercise after the other); rest 1 minute and then repeat entire circuit once or twice.

No.	Exercise	Page No.	Reps/Time
DAY 3			**FOCUS: CORE POWER AND STABILITY**
1	Medicine Ball Overhead Sit-Up	94	6 to 10
2	Medicine Ball Woodchopper	92	6 to 10
3	Swiss Ball Jackknife	72	10 to 12
4	High Chair Scissors	114	10 to 12

Perform exercises as a circuit (one exercise after the other); rest 1 minute and then repeat entire circuit once or twice.

14-Day Ab Sculpting Workout #1: Weeks 3 & 4

SPECIAL INSTRUCTIONS FOR WEEKS 3 & 4

- Perform three ab workouts each week. Incorporate two to three total-body strength workouts and two to three days of interval cardio in your program.
- Start with a general warm-up and then proceed to the Ab Warm-Ups (pages 24 to 39) before beginning these workouts.
- On Day 2, increase the weight you use for the Cable Woodchoppers and the Suitcase Dead Lifts from what you used in Weeks 1 & 2. But make sure the amount of weight you do use isn't so heavy that it compromises your form.

DAY 1			FOCUS: CORE STABILITY
No.	Exercise	Page No.	Reps/Time
1	Slow Sit-Up	46	10 to 12
2	Swiss Ball Bridge	84	30 to 60 seconds

Perform these two exercises as a circuit; rest 1 minute and then repeat circuit once or twice.

1	Medicine Ball Woodchopper	92	10 to 12 on each side
2	Swiss Ball Cobra	76	10 to 12

Perform these two exercises as a circuit; rest 1 minute and then repeat circuit once or twice.

DAY 2			FOCUS: CORE STRENGTH
No.	Exercise	Page No.	Reps/Time
1	Slant Board Reverse Crunch	108	10 to 12
2	Low to High Cable Woodchopper	102	6 to 8 on each side

Perform these two exercises as a circuit; rest 1 minute and then repeat circuit once or twice.

1	Knee-In	52	10 to 12
2	Suitcase Dead Lifts	124	6 to 8 on each side

Perform these two exercises as a circuit; rest 1 minute and then repeat circuit once or twice.

DAY 3			FOCUS: CORE POWER AND STABILITY
No.	Exercise	Page No.	Reps/Time
1	Medicine Ball Overhead Sit-Up	94	6 to 10
2	Medicine Ball Woodchopper	92	6 to 10

Perform these two exercises as a circuit; rest 1 minute and then repeat circuit once or twice.

1	Swiss Ball Jackknife	72	10 to 12
2	High Chair Scissors	114	10 to 12

Perform these two exercises as a circuit; rest 1 minute and then repeat circuit once or twice.

14-Day Ab Sculpting Workout #1: Weeks 5 & 6

SPECIAL INSTRUCTIONS FOR WEEKS 5 & 6

- Perform three ab workouts each week. Incorporate two to three total-body strength workouts and two to three days of interval cardio in your program.
- Start with a general warm-up and then proceed to the Ab Warm-Ups (pages 24 to 39) before beginning these workouts.
- Start adding or increasing the weight you used during Weeks 3 & 4. For instance, use a heavier medicine ball for the Kneeling Throw or do Supermans with light ankle and wrist weights. The weight should be heavy enough so that you can just complete the reps but not heavy enough to compromise your form.

DAY 1			FOCUS: STRENGTH AND EXPLOSIVE POWER
No.	Exercise	Page No.	Reps/Time
1	Knee-In	52	10 to 15
2	Swiss Ball Oblique Crunch	66	10 to 15
3	Medicine Ball Kneeling Throw	90	4 to 7
4	Supermans	118	4 to 7

Perform exercises as a circuit; rest 1 minute and then repeat entire circuit once or twice.

DAY 2			FOCUS: ROTATIONAL POWER
No.	Exercise	Page No.	Reps/Time
1	Medicine Ball Woodchopper	92	4 to 7
2	Crunch with Lateral Flexion	44	10 to 15
3	Vacuum	60	10 to 15

Perform exercises as a circuit; rest 1 minute and then repeat entire circuit once or twice.

DAY 3			FOCUS: CORE STABILITY
No.	Exercise	Page No.	Reps/Time
1	Swiss Ball Praying Mantis	86	10 to 15
2	Windshield Wipers	54	4 to 7
3	Overhead Squats	120	8 to 10

Perform exercises as a circuit; rest 1 minute and then repeat entire circuit once or twice.

14-Day Ab Sculpting Workout #2: Weeks 1 & 2

SPECIAL INSTRUCTIONS FOR WEEKS 1 & 2

- Perform three ab workouts each week. Incorporate two to three total-body strength workouts and two to three days of interval cardio in your program.
- Start with a general warm-up and then proceed to the Ab Warm-Ups (pages 24 to 39) before beginning these workouts.
- For any exercise that requires weight, use one heavy enough so that you can just complete the required number of reps with good form.

DAY 1			FOCUS: CORE STABILITY
No.	Exercise	Page No.	Reps/Time
1	V-Up	50	10 to 15
2	Swiss Ball Praying Mantis	86	10 to 15
3	Bicycles	58	10 to 15
4	Swiss Ball Cobra	76	10 to 15

Perform exercises as a circuit; rest 1 minute and then repeat entire circuit once or twice.

DAY 2			FOCUS: CORE STABILITY
No.	Exercise	Page No.	Reps/Time
1	Low-to-High Cable Woodchopper	102	10 to 15
2	Swiss Ball Jackknife	72	10 to 15
3	Swiss Ball Crunch with Cross Body Leg Lift	82	10 to 15

Perform exercises as a circuit; rest 1 minute and then repeat entire circuit once or twice.

DAY 3			FOCUS: ROTATIONAL STRENGTH & CORE STABILITY
No.	Exercise	Page No.	Reps/Time
1	Slow Sit-Up	46	10 to 15
2	Medicine Ball Kneeling Throw	90	10 to 15
3	Windshield Wipers	54	10 to 15
4	Suitcase Dead Lifts	124	10 to 15

Perform exercises as a circuit; rest 1 minute and then repeat entire circuit once or twice.

14-Day Ab Sculpting Workout #2: Weeks 3 & 4

SPECIAL INSTRUCTIONS FOR WEEKS 3 & 4

- Perform three ab workouts each week. Incorporate two to three total-body strength workouts and two to three days of interval cardio in your program.
- Start with a general warm-up and then proceed to the Ab Warm-Ups (pages 26 to 43) before beginning these workouts.
- Start adding or increasing the weight you used during Weeks 1 & 2. For instance, use a heavier weight for the Saxon Side Bends or do Hanging Leg Raises with light ankle and wrist weights. The weight should be heavy enough so that you can just complete the reps but not heavy enough to compromise your form.

DAY 1			FOCUS: CORE STABILITY
No.	Exercise	Page No.	Reps/Time
1	Swiss Ball Pass Off	78	10 to 15
2	Lateral Bridge	48	8 to 12
3	Twisting Pulse-Up	56	8 to 12
4	Supermans	118	8 to 12

Perform exercises as a circuit; rest 1 minute and then repeat entire circuit once or twice.

DAY 2			FOCUS: CORE STABILITY
No.	Exercise	Page No.	Reps/Time
1	High Chair Scissors	114	10 to 15
2	Saxon Side Bends	106	8 to 12
3	Swiss Ball Circle Crunch	68	10 to 15

Perform exercises as a circuit; rest 1 minute and then repeat entire circuit once or twice.

DAY 3			FOCUS: CORE STABILITY
No.	Exercise	Page No.	Reps/Time
1	Swiss Ball Corkscrew Crunch	70	10 to 15
2	Hanging Leg Raises	110	8 to 12
3	Cable Crunch	104	8 to 12
4	Unilateral Romanian Dead Lift	126	8 to 12

Perform exercises as a circuit; rest 1 minute and then repeat entire circuit once or twice.

14-Day Ab Sculpting Workout #2: Weeks 5 & 6

SPECIAL INSTRUCTIONS FOR WEEKS 5 & 6

- Perform three ab workouts each week. Incorporate two to three total-body strength workouts and two to three days of interval cardio in your program.
- Start with a general warm-up and then proceed to the Ab Warm-Ups (pages 26 to 43) before beginning these workouts.
- Start adding or increasing the weight you used during Weeks 3 & 4. For instance, use a heavier weight for the Overhead Squats and the Unilateral Romanian Dead Lifts. The weight should be heavy enough so that you can just complete the reps but not heavy enough to compromise your form.

DAY 1			FOCUS: CORE POWER AND STABILITY
No.	Exercise	Page No.	Reps/Time
1	Swiss Ball Bridge	84	60 seconds
2	Swiss Ball Crunch	64	10 to 15
3	Medicine Ball Bicycle	96	4 to 7
4	Overhead Squats	120	4 to 7

Perform exercises as a circuit; rest 1 minute and then repeat entire circuit once or twice.

DAY 2			FOCUS: CORE STRENGTH
No.	Exercise	Page No.	Reps/Time
1	Medicine Ball Overhead Sit-Up	94	4 to 7
2	Slant Board Reverse Crunch	108	10 to 15
3	Low-to-High Cable Woodchopper	102	4 to 7

Perform exercises as a circuit; rest 1 minute and then repeat entire circuit once or twice.

DAY 3			FOCUS: CORE STRENGTH AND STABILITY
No.	Exercise	Page No.	Reps/Time
1	Hanging Oblique Raise	112	10 to 15
2	Slant Board Reverse Crunch	108	10 to 15
3	Swiss Ball Figure Eights	74	10 to 15
4	Unilateral Romanian Dead Lifts	126	4 to 7

Perform exercises as a circuit; rest 1 minute and then repeat entire circuit once or twice.

Ab Workout To Go

This portable ab workout requires no equipment at all, just a bit of energy on your part. Now no matter where you are—visiting friends or family or holed up in a hotel room during a business trip—there's no excuse not to work out!

No.	Exercise	Page No.	Reps/Time
1	V-Up	50	8 to 10
2	Windshield Wipers	54	6 to 8 on each side
3	Slow Sit-Up	46	10 to 12
4	Lateral Bridge	48	8 to 10
5	Supermans	118	10 to 12

Perform exercises as a circuit; rest 1 minute and then repeat entire circuit once or twice.

About the Author

JAMES VILLEPIGUE has over 16 years of quality certified experience in the health and fitness industry as a nationally certified personal trainer with ACE and ISSA. He has received a degree from the New York College of Health Professions and is a massage therapist. James has also attended the accredited and highly acclaimed training school, the Institute for Professional Empowerment Coaching.

James was born on May 20, 1971, in Roslyn, New York. If you'd met James between the ages of 10 and 17, health and fitness would have been the last thing on your mind: At age 15 he weighed 250 pounds—and a thyroid deficiency was not to blame. James simply loved indulging in his favorite foods, as most Americans do.

James didn't know when to stop and certainly never considered the consequences of eating so much. Throughout high school, James was bullied and ridiculed to the point that he wanted to leave school permanently. Family members convinced him to stay and stick it out. James wasn't a tough kid and didn't like confrontation of any sort, but each day he was forced to defend himself mentally and physically.

Those tough years marked the turning point and the beginning of James's involvement with weight training.

James has now been involved with the health and fitness industries for more than a decade. He has certifications from the International Sports Sciences Association (ISSA) as a personal fitness trainer/counselor and from AFAA as a personal fitness trainer/counselor and weight room certified trainer. He was also appointed as a Strength and Conditioning Coach for the United States Karate Team. James also holds two U.S. patents and one Canadian Patent for a revolutionary piece of exercise/medical equipment called "Digiciser."

Throughout his career, James has kept up to date with the latest trends and rapid changes within the bodybuilding and fitness world. The adversity that once marked his life is not unlike the lives of so many teenagers and adults today. This, combined with his ability to create success out of his struggles, led him to dedicate his life to helping others make their fitness dreams and goals come true. When James thinks about his life now, he is grateful for the direction in which it has taken him, as he can now identify with anyone who struggles with eating disorders and adversity. Today, James Villepigue is a world-class fitness and bodybuilding trainer whose accomplishments have made him top in his class.

Resources

The following resource page presents a list of exciting web site addresses for your convenience. Here you will discover a plethora of useful information to help compliment your fitness life-style.

WWW.GETFITNOW.COM

Come join the fun and get interactive with the Web's most exciting fitness community.

WWW.MYCUSTOMWORKOUT.COM

The My Custom Workout programs offer the only fitness system designed to include absolutely *everyone*. Created to abolish the one-size-fits-all approach to fitness, the focus of the My Custom Workout programs is to customize individual and unique programs for each specific lifestyle.

WWW.ROCKINREPS.COM

Rockin-Reps is a self contained resistance training fitness system that uses a unique blend of music, time, and tempo that will help you achieve maximum fitness results. Through the use of our digitally mastered musical tracks and personal training directions, each program effortlessly guides you through the perfect workout and guarantees that you'll get the absolute best workout every workout session. In a nut shell, you will achieve the results that you never thought possible!

WWW.BICYCLEABS.COM

A recent study was conducted at the San Diego State University Bio Mechanics Lab and hosted by ACE (American Council on Exercise), searching for the most effective exercises for the abs. The results concluded that the number 1 exercise responsible for the highest recruitment of muscle activity was the Bicycle Maneuver. Ask any fitness expert and they will say the same thing: the bicycle is the most effective abs exercise there is! Now science and innovation have taken it a step further.

James Villepigue has developed a revolutionary abdominal machine which clearly has huge potential of becoming one of the most effective and best selling abdominal exercise devices in the marketplace. He is currently looking for qualified investors to be a part of this exciting endeavor. Please contact him for more details.